ADVANCE
Thai Yoga Massage

POSTURES AND ENERGY PATHWAYS
FOR HEALING

Kam Thye Chow

Healing Arts Press
Rochester, Vermont • Toronto, Canada

Healing Arts Press
One Park Street
Rochester, Vermont 05767
www.HealingArtsPress.com

Healing Arts Press is a division of Inner Traditions International

Note to the reader: *This book is intended as an informational guide. The remedies, approaches, and techniques described herein are meant to supplement, and not to be a substitute for, professional medical care or treatment. They should not be used to treat a serious ailment without prior consultation with a qualified health care professional.*

Library of Congress Cataloging-in-Publication Data is available
Chow, Kam Thye.
  Advanced Thai yoga massage : postures and energy pathways for healing / Kam Thye Chow.
    p. cm.
  Includes index.
  Summary: "Expand your Thai Yoga Massage practice with advanced postures and energy work to treat stress, back pain, headaches, and several other common conditions"—Provided by publisher.
ISBN 978-1-59477-427-0 (pbk.) — ISBN 978-1-59477-952-7 (e-book)

Printed and bound in the United States by the P. A. Hutchison Company

10 9 8 7 6 5 4 3 2 1

Text design and layout by Virginia Scott Bowman
This book was typeset in Sabon and Gill Sans with Delphin, Civet, and Gill Sans used as display typefaces

Photographs by Chirag Pandya, Studio Zoom Tech
Illustrations by Kam Thye Chow

To send correspondence to the author of this book, mail a first-class letter to the author c/o Inner Traditions • Bear & Company, One Park Street, Rochester, VT 05767, and we will forward the communication, or contact the author at **www.lotuspalm.com**.

Contents

FOREWORD

Cultivated Perception in Yoga and Thai Yoga Massage

Whether through dance, bodywork, or yoga, we can learn to cultivate our inner awareness. We sense the flow of our breath, any tension in our muscles, as well as the state of our mind and nervous system. As we refine this ability through ongoing practice, we come to trust what our senses tell us. Indeed in yoga philosophy, direct experience by someone who has systematically developed the ability to feel is considered the most reliable way of ascertaining what is true.

Masters of holistic healing traditions regularly use their rarefied perception to guide their lives as well as the healing approach they take with other individuals. Steady practitioners of yoga, for example, begin not only to be able to tell which yoga poses are good for them (or not so good!), but the mindfulness spreads to other areas of their lives. They may discern that a food that is supposed to be "healthy" makes them feel lethargic and bloated, and they do better without it. Or that a job that's high paying and well regarded leaves them feeling empty. Or that a particular type of therapeutic bodywork is profoundly relaxing to body and mind. That was my experience with Thai Yoga Massage; and in my yoga practice afterward, I was able to go more deeply than ever into several poses. I've seen similar synergy with such modalities as Rolfing and craniosacral therapy.

Modern medical science, of course, tends to discount such experiences. It believes that anecdotal evidence, as it calls all subjective experience as reported by individuals, is inherently unreliable. Expectations and selective memory can interfere with accurate reporting. True enough, but doctors tend to ignore direct experience almost entirely—even with patients who have cultivated embodied awareness for decades. Whenever possible, we physicians are supposed to recommend only those treatments that have been validated in randomized, placebo-controlled trials, no matter what people who have cultivated mindfulness for decades report.

Such experiments can indeed provide vital information, but due to ideological biases and financial incentives (most research is paid for by industry), many potentially useful treatments—including almost all systems of bodywork—never have been studied adequately. If you are suffering from a health condition, and ask your physician about something like Thai Yoga Massage, you are very likely to hear that "there isn't enough evidence to recommend it." But when scientific evidence is lacking, does it make sense to ignore—and deprive millions of patients—the potential benefits of modalities that experience suggests are safe and which thousands of embodied individuals report are effective?

Thai Yoga Massage came to me in 2004 when I lived as a scholar-in-residence at the Kripalu Center for Yoga and Health. It was in that picturesque setting in the Berkshire Mountains that I wrote much of my book *Yoga as Medicine.* Once I finished the first draft, for a couple of months I got to be a "kid in a candy store," taking any workshops I wanted, including a five-day training in Thai Yoga Massage. Over the course of the week, I got to both give and receive various treatments, and the benefits felt palpable. One thing that surprised me was the link to Ayurveda, the deep, indigenous healing tradition from India, which I integrate into my own practice and teaching of yoga and yoga therapy.

In *Advanced Thai Yoga Massage,* Kam Thye Chow explains how to go deeper into this healing art, and clearly delineates its connections to yoga and Ayurveda. With lucid explanations and excellent illustrations and photos, this book will help sincere practitioners refine their approach. A number of case histories demonstrate how Thai Yoga Massage, as part of a broader holistic approach, can be applied to clients suffering from a variety of disorders. But this is no cookbook. Kam Thye recognizes that there's more than one good way to help, and that people with similar symptoms sometimes need different approaches. Above all, he stresses that the practitioner's attitude, intention, compassion, and loving kindness may be the most important healing tools of all. His readers and their clients will be the beneficiaries of all the love, dedication, and embodied awareness that Kam Thye has put into writing this book.

NAMASTE,
TIMOTHY McCALL

Timothy McCall, M.D., is a board-certified internist, the medical editor of *Yoga Journal,* and the author of *Yoga as Medicine: The Yogic Prescription for Health and Healing* (Bantam). He lives in the San Francisco Bay Area and teaches workshops there and worldwide. He can be found on the web at www.DrMcCall.com.

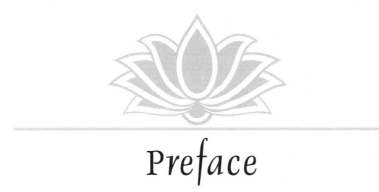

Preface

This book, two decades in the making, is the accumulation of all that I have learned in the study and practice of Thai Yoga Massage, beginning with six years at the side of my teacher, Asokananda, and continuing with fifteen more as founder of the Lotus Palm School in Montreal and teaching around the world. Like my own practice, this book is a reflection of Thai Yoga Massage—where it has come from and where it is heading.

So many things have changed about Thai Massage and the world. There was no Internet when I began my studies, and my teacher could communicate with students only through the postal service. There were very few schools, and Asokananda was writing the first foreign language book on the subject. Since then, terms such as "the global village" and "the world is flat"—meaning that technology is causing it to move faster than many of us can keep up with—have come into vogue, which says a lot about our rapidly globalizing world. We live on a planet where information, knowledge, and power are circulating more freely than ever before, and where people from all corners and walks of life are being given a fair chance to not only create and share their ideas but also to improve on some of the best ideas of yesterday. YouTube, Twitter, Facebook, and the blogosphere have fomented a massive rush to stake ground in the information world. The world has always moved this way, but what makes these days unique is the speed and universality with which all of these changes are taking place.

The growth and explosion of Thai Yoga Massage mirrors the frenetic pace at which our culture has been changing. In 1995 it seemed I was the only one teaching this art on the East Coast of North America. I struggled through many challenges to educate people on Thai Yoga Massage, so that there would be students to learn it and people to receive it. Nowadays most spas offer Thai Yoga Massage, every major city has at least one teacher, and thousands of people are hearing about it every day. It is impossible to keep track of all the people practicing and teaching Thai Yoga Massage.

This is an amazing development and a dream come true for anyone who loves Thai Yoga Massage. We have always known it is one of the best things you can do, both giving and receiving, and have felt in our heart of hearts that the more people who try it, the better the world becomes.

If there's a fly in the ointment, however, it's what to do now that this dream has come true. Has Thai Massage grown too much too soon? With so many different ways to teach and learn, and with no one standard format, questions continue to arise, such as, What is a Thai Massage? What is the traditional way of practicing? How do we preserve that, or keep up with the rising tide of change? I have often reflected on these questions over the years and this text will attempt to resolve at least some of them.

I will always be grateful and indebted to Asokananda for what he taught me. I sometimes reflect on my old friend and teacher who left the world much too soon, and I imagine the lively discussions we could have over this evolution—how to teach the art and speak to the current generation.

Asokananda adhered very closely to the way his teachers had taught him Thai Massage, because he strongly believed that his own teaching should be faithful to their tradition. I, however, am a practical person and have always thought that if this practice is to thrive and grow, people need to be able to learn it and continue to practice it on their own. It needs to make sense and be simple enough that anyone can pick it up and run with it, yet it needs to honor the essence of what I learned from my teacher. Looking deeply behind the postures and techniques, or using energy lines, what has always been the core truth of Thai Yoga Massage is metta—the physical application of loving kindness. The direction of my hand and all the meaning behind everything in the massage comes from this source. Universal compassion and kindness is the life force that gives meaning to energy and helps me to decide what postures to use. Everything else is a method and my job; my commitment and my art is to express it all in simple enough terms so that anyone can practice.

When I first started teaching in the West, I kept strongly to the form and method I had learned. I taught an introductory ten-day course in which students learned approximately three hours of Thai Yoga Massage postures and techniques that would set them on their way.

Sure enough, it didn't take long before I was affected by my students, particularly those I would eventually train to teach, and felt the creative pull to bring new insights into the practice. These changes were often about making sense of Thai Yoga Massage in the context of a new culture with a different audience. Students had different needs because of their Western body types, as well as the time they could dedicate to learning the art. Thus began the evolution of the Lotus Palm form.

I was among the first to split the ten-day course into shorter five-day courses, because I saw that it was too much for students to retain everything that was taught in ten consecutive days. The next major shift was to introduce the four fundamental basics at the core of the technique. These simple concepts that anyone can learn in an hour allow people to be their own teachers and flow gracefully from one posture to the next. In an effort to give students greater meaning to their work and effectively teach them about the energy in the body in the timeframe of a five-day course, I then introduced Ayurveda as the theoretical foundation of the practice.

Finally, in this book I have come back to the sen lines—the meridians through which life energy flows—to remodel them in a way that is easier to comprehend and put to good use. Ultimately all the pieces come together in order to use the postures, Ayurveda, sen lines, and even anatomy as a complete modality to address all manner of common ailments from a place of confidence, knowingness, and compassion.

These developments speak to one of my favorite sayings, which is, "Today's art is tomorrow's tradition." The creativity that comes with every Thai Yoga Massage, the infinite ways to combine postures, and the fact that there is an open spirit to the practice mean that it is all very much an art form that is open to interpretation. When people agree to use these techniques, this art form turns into a tradition, and in the space of fifteen years we have indeed established the Lotus Palm tradition that is practiced by thousands throughout the world.

In our modern world with its rapid evolution, everyone is an artist and traditions are repeatedly being built, taken apart, and reestablished. Traditions have become incredibly fluid and it is impossible to hold on to something that is, by definition, always changing. In the construct of time and reality, reality is now and time is the space. When we learn an art and freeze our knowledge in that space, we continue to practice and teach things in the ways our teachers taught us, and we hew to that as the greatest truth. However, we are constantly confronted by circumstances that ask us to cater to an ever-shifting reality. This is what we have been doing here, and this is what tradition means at Lotus Palm. Please use the information contained in this book and in all the books and your classes, but don't hold on too tightly to any of it.

Thai Yoga Massage is continuing to make itself known and we are constantly challenged to improve upon it, to present the art in its most professional way, and to continue to propagate this treasure in an ever-changing world. I, for one, am excited and just wish that I had my friend and teacher here to continue the discussion in this most exciting time. Asokananda, I dedicate this book to you.

Wishing you all a wonderful practice in yoga and Thai Yoga Massage,

Kam Thye Chow

Acknowledgments

This manual is a result of the help of many terrific people to whom I am indebted. Many thanks are extended to the following for their help and inspiration in bringing it to fruition:

The students of Thai Yoga Massage who inspire and challenge us to offer more techniques and courses to further your and our expertise

The many masters throughout the ages who have opened the doors for us to follow and contribute to the wealth of Thai Yoga Massage

The teachers and staff of Lotus Palm who have generously donated their time, particularly Shai Plonski, who has helped me put my thoughts into words, transcribing and editing the original manuscript, and Jyothi Watanabe, Sukha Wong, and Melaine Lecesne for their support, inspiration, and outstanding teaching

Julien Menard, an old soul in a young body, for all the support he has given Lotus Palm

Stephanie Golden, who has more passion for Thai massage than anyone else I know

Eleonore Piquet, my yoga instructor, who keeps me healthy

Deanne Pye and Kathleen Barbeau for keeping Lotus Palm strong and running while I am busy editing my book

Chirag Pandya who came to study Thai Yoga Massage and generously offered his services as a professional photographer

Guillaume Désilets for his support and love for Lotus Palm

Mirabai who is a beautiful yogini inside and out

Jasmine de Jager, who reminds me of Dakini, the Tibetan Sky Dancer

Dao Huan Chang, the model for the sen line photographs, who, coincidentally looks like the illustrations I drew before I met him

Jamaica Burns Griffin, my editor, and the staff at Inner Traditions who get a big thanks for doing a great job

A ghost from the past, Kailash, an old friend of mine who appeared out of the blue after twenty years

My sister, Chun Nooi, who was like a mother to me; she left the world too soon

And finally, my children, Keanu and Dana, who taught me so much about openheartedness and love: Daddy loves you more than you will ever know

❖

I arrived in Montreal and created Lotus Palm sixteen years ago; it has been a rewarding, satisfying, and challenging experience. We have managed to gain an international reputation as the foremost school of Thai Yoga Massage. This in many ways can be attributed to my teachers, students, and friends who contributed in the school's making. As the saying goes, timing is everything, and it is time for me to pass over leadership so that I can move on and continue my journey. It feels like I have come full circle. I took off on a tangent sixteen years ago, and now, in a simple way, I'm reconnecting back to my life where I began. That's where I'm most happy. So I want to thank you all from the bottom of my heart for this incredible Lotus Palm journey.

I couldn't be happier that Sukha Wong, my most senior teacher, is taking over ownership and leadership of Lotus Palm. Talk about a perfect fit. People who have such good organizational qualities and also embrace the spirit of metta are few and far between. One of Sukha's qualities that touches me most is her deep connection with her mother who taught her everything about kindness, survival, and how to face challenges with dignity. Her mother single-handedly brought up her children with little knowledge of English or Western culture; she's quite the woman. With this life experience, I have no doubt that Sukha will carry Lotus Palm to a greater level beyond our imagination. I wish her the best, and I will continue to support her and Lotus Palm and follow her leadership as a teacher and consultant.

Introduction

The practice of Thai Yoga Massage spans thousands of years, yet because it invokes our innate ability to heal and evolve, it is also the ideal twenty-first-century medicine. And because it affects not only the physical body but also more subtle emotional and spiritual planes, the results can seem truly miraculous.

In Thailand, Thai Yoga Massage practitioners have long been an integral part of the indigenous medical cultural system. The great masters are renowned for curing any number of illnesses, and people seek out a massage healer just as commonly as those in the West go to a medical doctor. In Thailand I've seen with my own eyes how this work helps people recover from crippling injuries, strokes, and even some who believe they are possessed by certain spirits.

As a practitioner in a Western setting, one is faced with the question of how to replicate that success and satisfaction in a different culture. The nature of the work, the expectations of clients for what constitutes a "great" massage, and people's intrinsic belief systems are all quite different from what is encountered in Thailand, challenging the Western practitioner to attain similar levels of excellence.

What's more, despite thousands of years of success stories that surround the practice, Western science insists that it is illogical for massage to be used to help cure so many of these illnesses. So the question persists: How does it all work? And how can it be made to work here?

IN A WORD: METTA

At the heart of Thai Yoga Massage and embodied in everything we do is the power of metta, or loving-kindness. Metta cannot be examined under a microscope, yet it is the greatest motivating power and is found in every cell of our bodies and the universe. Tapping into this spirit is the secret to every great treatment. Metta is the nourishment that feeds your ability.

One of the most radical teachings of the Buddha concerns the spirit of metta, that metta is not only about being pleasant or doing selfless work. It is a deeper understanding of the interdependency of all beings toward a shared purpose: to reach a state of true happiness.

As a physical application of loving-kindness, Thai Yoga Massage brings the spirit and benefits of meditation into a practical application and therefore allows people to be touched profoundly. It creates the necessary conditions for invoking the body's innate pranic healing power, both as therapist and client. At its best, it is part of a self-empowering healing system. For Thai Yoga Massage therapists, mastering this wonderful practice is a lifelong pursuit that is shared and passed down through the ages.

In understanding this path, one must realize that the structured methods of learning and the techniques, logic, and sequencing can bring you only to the door of mastership, but to truly attain such a level of practice requires strong faith. The great lesson to be learned is to eventually have complete trust in your ability to live in the present moment and be willing to let go of all you know. This skill is called "living the form of formlessness." From here you can tap into the vast reservoir of wisdom and energy that has been revealed to the masters throughout the ages. One of the great benefits of practicing at such an advanced level is that one's power of touch—with all parts of the body—is unlocked in every moment, and this knowledge can be used to listen to the body and create the essential massage experience. There is no outward test that indicates when you have reached this state, rather there is the inner certitude of tapping into and embracing the power of metta.

CREATING A GREAT THAI YOGA MASSAGE

The masters of Thailand practice therapeutic healing in a manner that is different from the approach used for general massage. It often focuses on certain areas and conditions of the body and is dynamically firmer—stronger and deeper. When practicing in the West, however, you must use much more caution to ensure that the massage isn't tortuous, and yet you must continue to work with the firm hand of metta.

Although your path is very much a personal journey, you can receive help by understanding that a great session has several essential components—meditation, body mechanics, and palpation or touch techniques—each of which is equally important.

Meditation

Pichet and Chaiyuth, two famous contemporary Thai healers, were asked in an interview, "Can meditation and devotion help you in your massage?" Chaiyuth's answer to that, in fractured English, was, "Yes! I talk to the Buddha every day. Every day, every day I talk to the Buddha." Pichet responded, "Yes I do, ah ah ah ah ah." Both answers remind us that these healers are devoted to meditation and the spirit of the Buddha. The inspiration for healing comes through the art of listening, being mindful, and working from the heart. Through your ability to have focused attention, it's almost as though the spirit of loving-kindness is doing the work and you become the vehicle, expressing it through your hands.

If meditation is not involved in the treatment, the experience often becomes mechanical. It literally doesn't draw inspiration. You will continue to be a beginner of the massage, waiting for the time when you can become a masterful healer. Tuning yourself to mindfulness is essential to completing a Thai Yoga Massage treatment.

Consider this quote from Bob Dylan: "I might look like I'm moving but I'm still on the inside." In other words, an open heart and deep listening are essential for opening up the possibilities of healing. Carrying this energy into your practice gives you the ability to create the physical elements of your Thai Yoga Massage treatment.

Body Mechanics

Excelling with your body mechanics is the first step in bringing forward your internal light. One of the reasons so many people are first attracted to Thai Yoga Massage is because it is a practice as well as a way to make a living, and done well, it is as beneficial for the giver as it is for the receiver. Part of becoming a master means that more and more you will apply the lessons you learn through the practice to your everyday life. Your stances, your rhythm, and your attention to detail are all-encompassing.

Palpation and Touch Techniques

In this aspect the application of Thai Yoga Massage as practiced in Thailand may differ greatly from the way it's practiced in the West. Always, your skill and the way you touch your clients must be accompanied by an understanding of culture and expectations.

In Thailand, Thai Yoga Massage is deeply connected to the spirit of shamanic healing, and sometimes contemporary masters embody the spirits of great healers, such as Hanuman, the Hindu monkey god. When the trance state takes over, these masters have been witnessed jumping up and down on tables and even licking the recipient's ear like a monkey. But even more to the point is the expectation in Thailand of "no pain, no gain." Thai Yoga Massage can be very intense and very often if the tears are flowing, you know you are getting to the root of the issue. However, the culture of massage in the West is quite different; the goal is often a soothing approach with a relaxing result, so rather than trying to emulate the Thai masters on the surface level, go deeper to create the experience with a Western sensibility. You can reach the same state of excellence when you bring your full intention of metta into your work and "listen" to the recipient's body. Listening is something you do not only with your ears but with your whole being.

This is the magic elixir that stirs the drink. You must be able to develop this listening capacity equally well with your hands, feet, and knees. How does listening work? From the very first moments the recipient is continually relaying messages through the body, so this time window is essential for setting up the proper therapeutic space and establishing a sense of trust, communication, metta, and friendship that will carry you through the session.

In the very first instants you can discover the client's likes and dislikes, as well as how receptive he is to your movements. Our experience shows that practitioners often bring this intent listening to the beginning and end of the massage, but there is a tendency to start to drift during the middle stages of the treatment. In fact, this is the greater challenge, as on an energetic level you are so often tested before a deeper healing potential is revealed. It's the ability to remain serene, balanced, and non-judgmental throughout the entire massage that remains key. When this is maintained you can continue to adjust, remain flexible, and palpate with thumbs, fingers, hands, elbows, feet, knees, and your whole body. You can choose the techniques best suited for every moment for both practitioner and receiver. And you can take the potential of a Thai Yoga Massage beyond the physical to the emotional and spiritual levels of bliss.

The test of mindfulness as it's related to listening is therefore vital, because when you can reach this space, you can quiet the ego. You are no longer doing what you think is best but what the recipient is asking for from his or her deeper core, allowing you both to tap into the healing capacity of this individual body. Ideally, as you develop a rapport, you can then begin to introduce stretches, breathwork, and lifestyle changes the client can incorporate into her everyday life.

If the situation is therapeutic, it's recommended to schedule regular visits—weekly is most common—yet give the client a chance to integrate the effects of the massage for a few days before continuing with the next treatment. And as you customize your massage, it is perfectly acceptable to focus on the most problematic areas for two or three sessions at a time, but it's also important to remember the holistic foundation of Thai Yoga Massage and return to a full-body treatment every three or four sessions. I recommend that treatment plans begin with a six-session weekly wellness program, to be followed by a monthly tune-up.

CREATING A GREAT THAI YOGA MASSAGE PRACTICE

Creating a fulfilling practice requires two important qualities: passion and compassion. I would like to share a couple of stories from members of the Lotus Palm community that illustrate this.

Recently one of our students, Brian, participated in a round-table discussion led by a medical doctor exploring alternative ways to treat a woman with fibromyalgia. Massage experts from different fields of expertise included a polarity expert who talked about balancing the person's energy, a Reiki expert who discussed raising the person's vital energy, and a deep-tissue therapist who focused on releasing the trigger points. The doctor noticed Brian had not been contributing much to the conversation, and so he asked his opinion. Brian's response took everyone off guard when he said he thought the patient could be best helped through kind, compassionate touch. The doctor was so impressed that he approached Brian later to personally request a massage treatment. Why is this a success? Because we must always remember that our treatment comes from the heart.

I have many success stories of our teachers and students offering massage to aid in the cure of dependency of drug addiction, debilitating pain, and much more. One of the more inspiring of these comes from a client being treated for an undiagnosed energy deficiency. Although in many ways the client appeared healthy, she had long suffered from very low energy, being constantly tired of mind and body. This unremitting in-between stage of health and illness had been very frustrating throughout her life, as it was difficult for people around her to take her complaints seriously. She'd been turned away from experts more times than she could count. Yet when the treatments began it was clear that her vital energy was severely low and blocked; she could barely move her legs and was constantly resisting every movement. After just eight weeks of treatment, she came out of a massage with her eyes brimming with unbelievable joy, feeling like the puppet Pinocchio who could suddenly walk and talk. A lifetime of frustration began to recede as she started to awaken and feel her body as truly alive.

It's these types of experiences that continue to recur in our personal journeys as teachers, therapists, and even patients, and feed our faith in metta. They motivate us to build on our practice by passing on some of these discoveries to you.

WHAT TO EXPECT FROM THIS MANUAL

Our first goal is to help facilitate and further develop the master within each therapist. Our intention is to initiate and develop the form of formlessness. Up to this point in your development (with my books *Thai Yoga Massage* and *Thai Yoga Therapy for Your Body Type*) I have presented new poses as part of a logical flow that moves from sitting, through feet and legs, until finally reaching the head. Here I will be encouraging you to develop the flow and transitions that best speak to you, in order to encourage the highest result with your client.

We will discuss some determining factors, including:

- What your client brings to the mat, including presenting issues and abilities
- What you bring to the mat, including your personal skill set and presenting issues
- The intuitional moment-to-moment awareness

We will explore all of the sen lines in depth, including the full running of the lines, landmarks, properties, and how to use them in the massage.

We will be adding new postures to your practice and examining eight case studies of some of the more common ailments we encounter. And you will explore treatment plans that integrate all the parts of your Thai Yoga Massage knowledge.

I wish you lifelong enjoyment and skillful practice of the "Buddha's medicine."

OM SHANTI

The Heart of the Lotus Palm System

The primary intention of the Lotus Palm system of Thai Yoga Massage is to give you the tools to become your own teacher. Our goal is always to introduce postures and create a familiarity so that the inner sense is strong. You should be able to answer the question, "Why does this feel right?" Or conversely, when not using good mechanics, "Why does it feel wrong?"

To better assist with this process, the foundation of every course we teach and of your practice is the four basics: Meditation and metta, stances, rhythmic rocking, and touch techniques. As your practice develops, these four basics become more important than ever. As you develop the form of formlessness, a deep-rooted understanding of the four basics will steer you in the right direction and create smooth transitions from one posture to the next, ensuring that you use your body to the best and safest of your abilities.

1. MEDITATION AND METTA

Much has been said about the importance of incorporating meditation and metta into your work. Suffice it to say that this is the foundation from which your massage flows. One of the ways to incorporate it into the massage is through breath work. The most common breathing techniques used in the massage are:

Mindful breath: Being aware of your inhale and exhale, remaining present throughout.

Guided breath: Asking your client to inhale, and then working with the exhale to take her deeper into a stretch.

Double breath: Similar to the guided breath, but the steps are repeated for those who can go deeper into the stretch.

Forced or induced breath: Most commonly used when you work on the back. When you press on the back you can control the rhythm of the breath. You are literally forcing the recipient to exhale when you press down and creating an inhale when you release. As such you can gradually work deeper and longer with every exhale, expanding the recipient's optimal limits a shade or two.

Synchronized breathing: Most commonly used during the abdominal part of the massage. This is the one time when the practitioner and recipient can come together to share a breath naturally. It is used to calm the energy and nurture a sense of trust while working on the emotional center of the body.

2. STANCES

There are a number of stances that are appropriate for a practitioner of Thai Yoga Massage. Ideally you will flow smoothly from one to the other in the course of a treatment.

Diamond Stance

- ◆ Kneeling and sitting on the heels
- ◆ Back straight, eyes looking forward

Variation: Sitting on your heels with toes tucked under

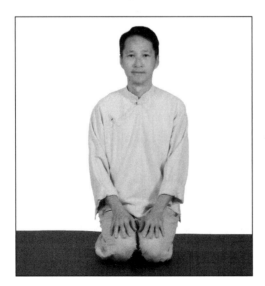 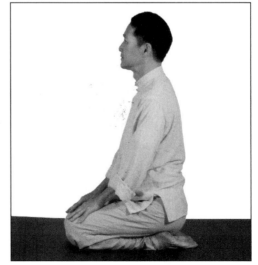

Open Diamond Stance

◆ Similar to Diamond but with knees separated

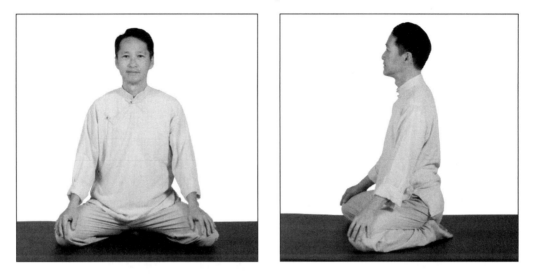

Variation: Tuck toes under while still sitting on your heels. This allows you to raise your stance to accommodate size differences between you and your client. For example, if you are much shorter than your client, this variation allows you to find the right height to comfortably perform the neck massage.

Kneeling Diamond Stance

◆ Bringing the knees slightly together and coming up on your knees

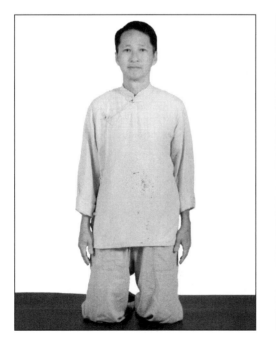
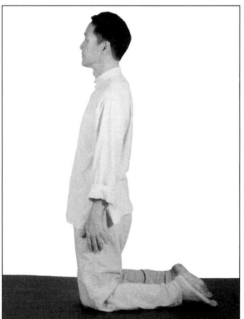

Warrior Stance

♦ Raise your right knee up and place your right foot flat on the floor at a right angle to your body. The knee and foot should line up, so that the knee doesn't extend beyond the toes.

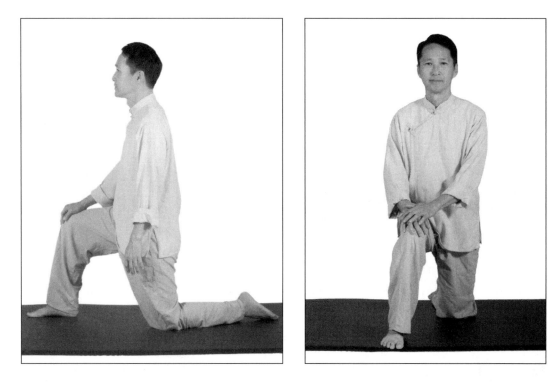

Variation: Gliding Warrior is used to make adjustments in distance between you and the recipient. You can move in Warrior by extending your front leg and then sliding your back leg along the mat, pulling the body forward.

It's important to remember that what you do with your front leg needs an equal response from the back leg, and vice versa, so that you remain balanced and strong with each movement.

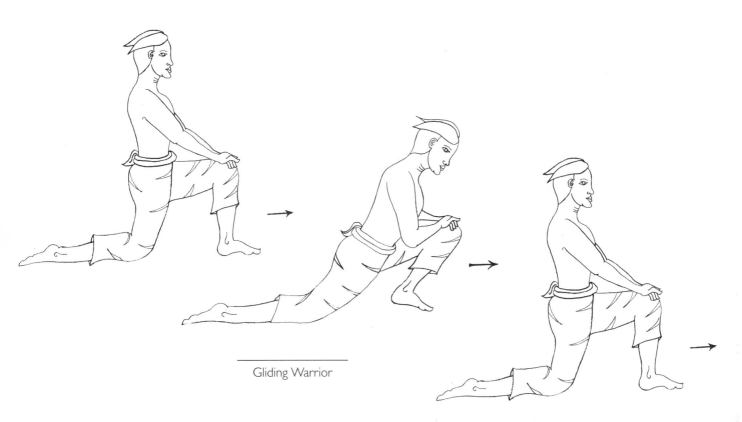

Gliding Warrior

Open Warrior Stance

♦ Similar to Warrior, but the raised knee is shifted to the side with the hips facing straight ahead. The knee is again lined up above the foot, only this time it is to the side.

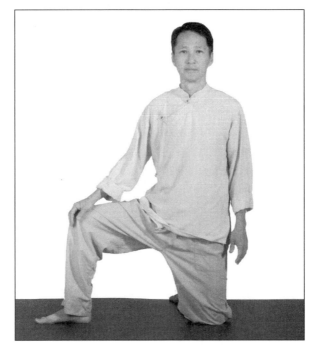

Archer Stance

♦ From Warrior stance, curl your back toes under, sit back on your back heel, and bring your front foot close, so that you are resting on your front toes. One knee is always anchored on the mat while the other is up.

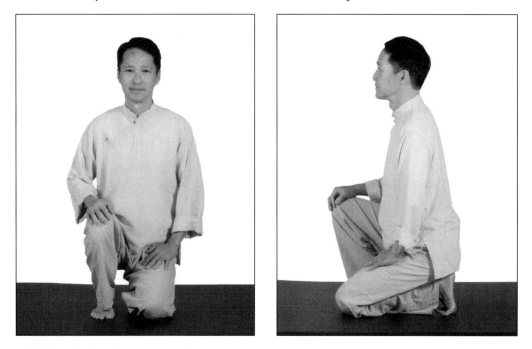

Open Archer Stance

♦ Similar to Archer stance, but open your front leg to the side.

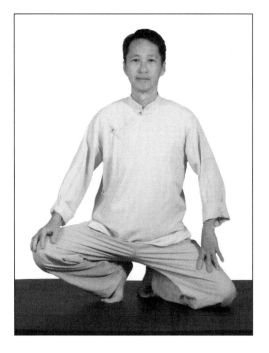
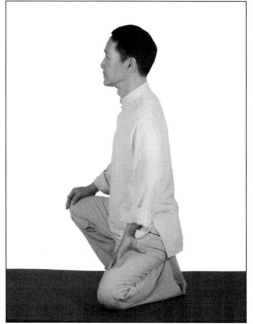

Tai Chi Stance

- ♦ Step straight up.
- ♦ Bring the back foot even with the back of the forward foot and step forward into Tai Chi stance.

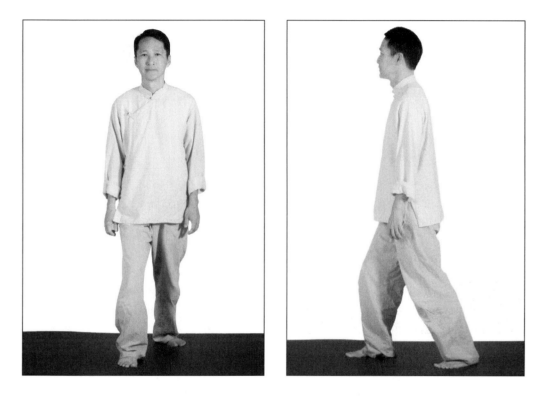

3. RHYTHMIC ROCKING

Rhythmic rocking is truly one of the most important aspects of the massage. It establishes the tempo that is carried through the entire treatment.

The rocking also creates a nurturing and relaxing motion that helps with the flow of the massage. It is also the means by which you alter pressure and momentum and create leverage during the massage.

There are three rhythmic rocking techniques:

Forward Rock

- ♦ Sit in Diamond stance moving forward and back.
- ♦ There is a slight nuance involved. When moving forward, the chin is slightly raised, and when moving backward, the chin is slightly tucked to ensure a straight spine. The moving forward and back is done from the hips so that the spine doesn't curve.

Side to Side (Bamboo Rock)

- Sit in an Open Diamond stance and rock your shoulders side to side like bamboo trees in the wind. Your head should follow the spine.

Whirlpool Rock

- In Open Diamond stance, rotate your upper body first in one direction, then the other.
- Begin slowly, then gradually increase the size of the rotations.

4. TOUCH TECHNIQUES

Touch techniques are critical to an outstanding massage experience. All contact with the recipient involves touch, whether putting the recipient into a stretch or using your hands, arms, knees, and feet to provide that incredible feeling of being massaged.

The art of touch in massage is similar to what a deep sea diver does when searching for treasures at the bottom of the ocean. In order to find them he has to put attention into his hands and fingers, because they become his eyes. In our case, the body's hidden treasures can be found in unlocking sore muscles, tension spots, and tired areas where they are exposed as ripples, ropes, golf balls, stiffness, and more. The art of palpation is learning how to touch with awareness and listen to the quality of the body.

Body Talk

An expert Thai Yoga Massage therapist is able to gauge exactly where to stop in a stretch or touch so that it feels good. The "pain" the recipient sometimes feels is positive and therapeutic. It never becomes uncomfortable or torturous because it is done through awareness, practice, and listening to what the recipient is communicating. That information is all found in the subtle language of nonverbal communication.

To bring someone into a stretch, find the limit of his range of motion and hold him there. With repetition, the body tends to respond and relax, and it can be brought to a new limit.

A Thai Yoga Massage stretch is deep and dynamic. As you learn to speak this language—and generally at various points throughout your massage—check in with your recipient as to comfort level. If you feel resistance or the body accommodating*

Accommodating means the recipient will shift his body to relieve discomfort. For example, if you lift the recipient's arm above his head and pull it backward, it will get to the point where the hip and the back will begin to move forward to accommodate.

then you know you have gone too far. You have gone much too far when the muscles tremble. The best stretch puts the person at that space just before resistance where there is no need for accommodation.

General Rules for Touch

Although there are a number of different types of touch and different ways to approach them, there are basic rules that support safety and a positive experience.

Use a Gradual Approach

- For stretching: Do not take the person directly to his maximum. Hold back, and if you feel the muscles release, you can move the stretch slightly deeper, one step at a time.
- For massage: Do not go directly to the deepest part of the muscle. You always want to prepare the area for deeper work; therefore begin with palming before using other parts of your body.
- You do not have to bring a person to the maximum stretch or touch the deepest part of the muscle in order for benefits to be felt. It is a holistic approach and the whole massage is benefiting the recipient in countless ways. You want to stretch only as far as your body, your recipient's body, and your knowledge of safe practice allows.

Find Your Source of Pressure

- The pressure comes from your center, belly, or core.
- Whatever part of your body you use, always continue to stay aware of how you can use your whole body to help provide pressure and to support you in your touch or stretch.
- A general rule of arms extended, back straight, and chin up helps to support this principle.
- Do not lock your elbows.
- Keep bringing attention to your back. All parts should be straight (although not stiff), extending from the bottom to the very top.

Save Your Wrists, Hands, and Thumbs

- ♦ Palm using the fleshy part closest to your wrist.
- ♦ Avoid hyperextending your wrist (that is, at an angle of more than 70°).
- ♦ Thumb using the fleshy part in the center of the pad.
- ♦ Do not put more than half of your body weight onto your thumb.

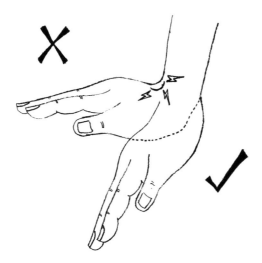

Wrist-saving technique

Avoid Repetitive Strain

- ♦ Vary palming by using soft fists.
- ♦ Reduce thumbing by using elbows, rolling pin, knees, and feet.

With practice you will continue to develop awareness and comfort using all parts of your body. In this way it is entirely possible and recommended to give a massage that responds to your recipient's every wish without using your thumbs and greatly reducing the use of your palms.

THAI YOGA MASSAGE SIGNATURE TOUCH TECHNIQUES

Palm Hopping

About 70 percent of the pressure is applied through the heel of the hand; 30 percent is spread throughout the rest of the hand and fingers. Sit in Open Diamond stance and rock forward onto your palms. Pause, and then rock back releasing the pressure. Shoulders should not extend beyond your wrists.

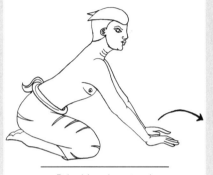

Palm Hopping, step 1

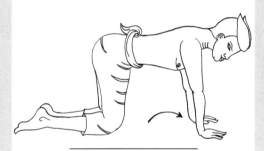

Palm Hopping, step 2

Palm Chasing Palm

In Open Diamond stance, first extend your right palm, applying pressure through a side-to-side rock. Then rock to your other side, applying pressure with the left palm.

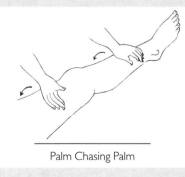

Palm Chasing Palm

THE THREE GEMS OF A SUCCESSFUL MASSAGE JOURNEY

The three gems of Thai Yoga Massage bring the stances to life so that you can personalize and combine them to find your most comfortable and effective position. They help create awareness of the slight adjustments required between every transition. Use the three gems to help you find better angles, so that you can use your body weight instead of forcing pressure through your hands, and to make those adjustments that turn Thai Yoga Massage into a graceful, flowing, energizing experience for you as well as the recipient.

Four-Wheel Drive

Just as the four wheels of a car need to be in good alignment in order for it to function optimally, so must your body's "four wheels": two shoulders and two hips. The general rule is that your four wheels should always be facing the same direction and facing your work, so when you move your upper body to apply a touch technique, it's important to also turn your lower half so that you can comfortably fall in with your work.

In single leg exercises, for example, you regularly need to adjust your body between most postures, or even during the postures as the direction of the recipient's leg changes or she relaxes into a stretch. Four-wheel drive reminds you to keep shifting your body along with your recipient, so that you can maximize the leverage of your body to effectively compress and apply pressure.

Steering Mechanism

Your ability to keep your four wheels in alignment depends on how smoothly you drive your car or body on all kinds of terrain. In this case, the steering wheel is your head and the steering column is your legs. Your head leads, and your legs should follow. As you move from posture to posture, always facing your work, your work is the point of contact where you intend to apply a touch technique. Begin by locating the work, and then steer your four wheels into alignment by adjusting your stance as necessary. This is especially true when moving into and out of all variations of Warrior and Archer stances. You fine tune your alignment by opening or closing your stance, gliding forward or back, wagging your tail, and knee walking.

Distancing

Maintaining a good distance is vital to using your body well. The common rule of "arms extended, back straight, chin up" means that it's important to find the right distance so that you can fall in properly with your body weight. Often there is a tendency when learning new postures to be too close to the recipient, especially when practicing foot and single-leg exercises. However, it's best to take care to move back, trust that you are supporting your client, and then fall in with your body.

KEYS TO A SAFE AND RESPECTFUL PRACTICE

We are all in the practice and the business of wanting to help our recipients and give the greatest massage possible. While it is commendable to want to give everything you've got and then some, this very powerful wish can also lead over time to injury and compromise the safety of your body and hands. You must remember to ask yourself how much good you would be able to provide if you were unable to practice your craft.

A second common occurrence is to become so focused on the massage that you forget to pay attention to your recipient. This could mean brushing up too close with your intimate body parts, or even massaging with too much pressure or putting someone in too great of a stretch. It is important to remember—and internalize into every cell—that the first rule to a successful massage is respect. This applies to you as much as it applies to the recipient.

Your first consideration is always your recipient's physical and emotional boundaries. There are several ways to maintain this awareness throughout the massage:

- Check in at the beginning regarding general health and any physical limitations, including follow-up questions from previous sessions. If the recipient mentions something, ask for more specific details. For example, if she mentions her left shoulder is sore, ask her to show you exactly where. Similarly, ask her to move her shoulder in all directions so you have a clear understanding of her flexibility and movement before putting her into a stretch.
- Check in for pressure and comfort a few times throughout the massage. A good time to ask is at the beginning, as well as when the receiver turns over.
- Use props liberally. Pillows, blankets, bolsters, and meditation cushions have the great benefit of adding comfort to the massage as well as helping you to maintain space between your and your recipient's bodies.
- Avoid any hint of sexual proximity, especially in the breast or genital area. Thai Yoga Massage moves the body in three dimensions and into all shapes. Therefore, you need to take extra care to avoid coming too close to your recipient. For example, when you transition your recipient into the Tree pose, it is normal to be right behind the knee. The next step is to palm the upper leg, and if you're not careful, it is possible that your groin will come very close to the recipient's knee,

so you need to shift to the side to avoid that contact. Be aware of similar possibilities and make any necessary adjustments to your massage, including using props to create proper space.

♦ Should your recipient experience an emotional release, it is important to be fully present for this and not avoid issues or be caught unprepared. Simply pause and allow the emotions to pass, while internally practicing metta and loving compassion. Once it passes the recipient can decide whether or not to continue.

♦ Follow the natural anatomy of your recipient's body. For example, in Knee to Shoulder, do not take the name literally! Let the recipient take the lead and allow the leg to open in whatever direction the hip wants to go. Similarly, the shoulder is the most mobile joint in the body; however, when your recipient is lying flat on the table, the shoulder is not able to make a 360° circle. Get to know the body and work within those limits. The focus of the massage is to work the muscles and avoid any direct pressure on bones. This is especially true of the spine, which is the main telecommunication system of the body.

Fine-Tuning Your Massage

Taking great care of yourself is fundamental to creating a thoroughly enjoyable experience and ensuring a long-lasting career. The four basics and the three gems are your teachers and frame every aspect of the massage, so continue to internalize them with every massage you give.

Other elements that will elevate your massage include:

♦ Avoid force or jerky movements. When placing your recipient in a posture or transitioning from one position to the next, use your body weight rather than muscular force. Work with rotations, for example the Helicopter, to help prepare your recipient for the deeper stretch to come, and to help eliminate resistance from one movement to the next.

♦ Practice all of your stances so that they become second nature. With proper alignment, including keeping your back straight and your head up, you will be able to maintain a good distance without your body feeling rigid, thus facilitating smooth and continuous movement.

♦ Move in a fluid manner by practicing rhythmic rocking techniques in all your stances throughout every part of the massage. Even the hand, head, and abdomen massage should include some feeling of movement. This graceful flow is the basis for an elegant and economic use of energy and helps prevent build-up of tension or fatigue. The table presents an immobile surface that takes some getting used to when incorporating a flow into your routine. However, with practice it becomes an extension of you. It is another wonderful tool that goes along with your body so that when you employ the dance of Thai Yoga Massage, the recipient feels the benefit of your full presence.

♦ Practice good personal hygiene. Wash your hands before and after a massage and keep your fingernails and toenails trimmed and clean. Wear clean, comfortable clothes that fit properly. Keep your massage area clean, including props and sheets. Keep hand sanitizer and tissues in your room.

Massage Pathways

The Sen Lines and Marmas

The gopichand, also known as a gopiyantra, is an ancient Indian instrument that consists of a stick, a cone, and a string. It makes an enchanting natural sound that often sets the rhythm and background for singing, chanting, or reciting poems, and it is so simple that with some practice and discipline, just about anyone can play it.

The same can be said about the art of sen energy-line work, which is also based on intuition and natural rhythm. According to the yoga philosophy upon which Thai Yoga Therapy is based, there are 72,000 energy lines running through our bodies. Of these lines, ten are of key importance to Thai Yoga Massage. These lines, known as the sip sen, connect many of the marmas, or pressure points, throughout the body. Massaging the sen promotes the free flow of prana through these important energy hubs.

In Thailand, the teaching of sen energy lines differs according to geography and region. Some of the most respected schools teach multiple interpretations of the same energy-line system; even within the same village one might find two masters teaching different body locations and healing properties for the same sen lines. On the surface this may seem contradictory and confusing, but the healing results of these masters cannot be denied. We have observed these healers enter into a deep meditative state that transcends the limitations of any physical landmark or location; they feel the location of the lines through an intuitive touch, loving-kindness, and a devotion to healing.

There are many interpretations of the sen energy-line locations, but with the correct intention and spirit, any devoted practitioner will be able to practice and master this system.

APPROACHING THE SEN LINES

In Thai Yoga Massage the energy lines are worked through muscle palpation, assisted yoga *asanas,* and stretches. Working with a relaxed and playful energy will encourage you to open up to your intuition. For example, when you bring a person into cobra, you can visualize the opening of the Sen Kalathari at the abdomen, through the chest, down the arms, and into the hands. Every individual has a unique body, and for that reason the exact pathways and locations of the lines run differently for each person. It is therefore impossible to apply a predetermined energy-line map to all of your clients. The knowledge of the sen energy-line system provides you with a strong theoretical base to begin your energy-line work, yet if you get stuck on following these details too rigidly, you run the risk of staying in your head and missing out on the true needs of the client. Energy-line work must be centered in the heart, not the intellect.

As you place your hands on your client in preparation for the sen energy-line work, notice the quality of your thoughts. At first you may find yourself thinking about the precise location of the lines as illustrated in this book, or perhaps as you learned them during a recent workshop. Over time, as your confidence builds, you should become less dependent on these supports and instead allow intuition to direct your work. Rather than referring to external resources that teach the general location of the lines, find yourself turning inward to listen to the energetic composition of each client. When approached in this way, sen energy-line work generates a deep state of relaxation and promotes centeredness and well-being for both client and practitioner.

The treatment properties discussed here are based on the teachings of my teacher Asokananda and his translation of ancient Thai texts. The demarcation of the lines comes from Asokananda and our teachers Chaiyuth and Pichet. They have been further modified by Lotus Palm to retain their potency but make them simpler to use in real-life situations. The accuracy and validity of these lines are subject to further research for their value and usability. Indeed, since Thai Yoga Massage has gone global and is receiving more attention than ever, the usefulness and effectiveness of the massage and all its parts will be more and more subject to analysis and understanding that will benefit all who love this massage form.

Why We Use Sen Lines

The sen lines are an integral part of a 2,500-year-old tradition, and although this theoretical approach cannot be fully explained, it has a powerful therapeutic effect. There are, in fact, many things that cannot be totally explained but are still useful. Perhaps in the current millennium science will have a full explanation of the sen lines, but even without an in-depth scientific study there is ample evidence showing that Thai Yoga Massage is effective, and that is partly because of the sen lines.

The interconnectedness of the body, energy, emotions, and intelligence—the cosmic flow—is very important. A toe belongs to you as much as your ears and eyes do. The body is constantly working in partnership to both absorb the wear and tear of daily life and propel us forward toward a better existence. If you injure your right hip, your back, ankle, and knee are just some of the areas where adjustments will be made to compensate. Similarly, if you are feeling incredible throughout your back and shoulders, this is bound to have a positive effect down your arms and hands. Therefore, it goes without saying that working on your toes can have a great effect on the ears. The sen lines guide us in how to make great use of this connection for a deeper therapeutic effect.

Thai Yoga Massage energy lines also have a valuable contribution to make to yoga. In yoga philosophy, Sushumna, Ida, and Pingala *nadis* (energy lines) are well recognized and taught. Even though 72,000 sen lines are referenced, it is primarily these three energy lines that are used in yoga. In Thai Yoga Massage we have seven more that come from a similar background that we can reintroduce into yoga. Many of the great Indian yogis have come to the West because they have the money and support of followers of the practice. As a result, many Indians are coming west to study yoga, and the same is true for Thai Yoga Massage.

There are ten primary sen lines in Thai Yoga Massage and some run in pairs, so they cover six principal routes along the body:

- Ittha/Pingkhala
- Thawari/Sahatsarangsi
- Lawusang/Ulangka
- Nanthakrawat/Khitchanna
- Kalathari
- Sumana

The sen lines are used on the physical body, but they touch and connect with all the subtle places of the human body.

The Kosha Bodies

According to yoga philosophy, everything in the universe is animated by an essential life force. The same vital energy we spoke of earlier in the discussion of metta is known as prana, and it manifests itself in different densities that are expressed through five layers, or kosha bodies: the physical body, annamaya kosha; the energetic body, pranamaya kosha; the mind body, manamaya kosha; the wisdom body, vijnanamaya kosha; and finally the blissful body, or anandamaya kosha.

Annamaya kosha. This is the physical body. It is the most gross, consisting of muscles, bones, and connective tissues, and the associated aches and pains.

Pranamaya kosha. This is the energetic body that breathes life into all corners of your body. Here is where you start to bridge the physical, that which you can see and that which is more subtle. However, there is also a physiological component, as it relates to parts of your system responsible for movement, namely the nervous, lymphatic, and endocrine systems.

Manomaya kosha. This is the mental body. It is your organizational, thinking, and reactive mind. It also involves your feelings and emotions.

Vijnanamaya kosha. This is the intellectual, or wisdom, body. This body takes the mental body one step further by being the framework for how you make decisions. Here you touch on the subconscious, environmental, and social conditioning and how it influences this body.

Anandamaya kosha. The blissful body is the most subtle body and is experienced when you are living in the present moment. It is the sense of contentment, joy, peace, and wonder that you feel when everything aligns, even for just a moment. It is where choice originates and life is lived when we are in greater alignment.

Obstructions in the flow of energy result in an insufficient supply of prana and cause imbalances in the kosha bodies, preventing us from being aware and living our bliss. All of the stretches and massage techniques used in a Thai Yoga Massage help to restore and improve the flow of vital energy throughout the body.

Using the Sen Lines

We usually work on sections of the body at a time. Very often we begin with a few stretches or articulations to warm up an area, proceed with palming or thumbing lines, and then finish up with more stretching to integrate the effects. Taking the feet as an example, we work on the sen lines of our choice with some combination of palming, thumbing, kneeing, and so on, and add yoga postures. When working on the feet, the order of postures or choosing to directly massage sen lines first versus postures is a personal choice based on a moment-to-moment awareness and personal interpretation. Once the feet are finished, move on to the next section, such as the legs, and continue in the same way.

The sen lines are worked through:

- Directed touch techniques of palming, thumbing, elbowing, kneeing, and walking
- Assisted yoga postures or stretching
- Directing the client's breath
- The therapist mentally directing his intention

In a stretch, how you position the body can have an important effect. For example, in the Row Boat, where you are holding the arms while walking up and down the back, the rotation of the shoulders changes the sen line on which you are working. When the shoulders are rotated so that the recipient's thumbs point downward, the recipient experiences the posture more through the top of the shoulders, down the top of the bicep forearm, and into the thumb. That is the running of Sen Sahatsarangsi and Thawari.

Turn the shoulders out slightly and the recipient feels it more down the center of the arm—Sen Kalathari.

Rotate the shoulders all the way out and the recipient feels it down the armpit all the way into the pinkie finger—Sen Ittha and Pingkhala.

Selecting the Appropriate Sen Line

If we ask ten accomplished Thai Yoga Massage therapists to massage a person with back pain, we will have ten very different massages with different emphasis on which energy lines to use. Yet as long as they each put their whole heart and effort into it, we will also end up with ten very effective Thai Yoga Massage sessions. That is the beauty of the practice. So it is important to remember that selecting energy lines is based equally on theory and intuition. The theory gives some meaning to the practice and is a foundation on which you can understand what you're doing so that you are free and able to trust your intuition. Therefore, anyone practicing with this kind of effort is right and no one is wrong.

At Lotus Palm, Kalathari is generally the main line we use, as well as the first line we teach, and the rest of the lines are often used in support of this line. Sen Kalathari runs along the principal arteries of the body acting as a second pump to the heart. It crosses through the emotional center and digestive center at the navel/small intestine, as well as reaching every extremity from the fingertips to the toes. Therefore, our sense of this line is that it runs deeply through all of the five koshas. You can use this energy line to relax the body deeply as well as to provide an energetic boost and circulation to all parts of the body. It is beneficial for vata, pitta, and kapha dosha types in the Ayurvedic system of body-mind composition.*

In our school we make the link between sen lines—where they travel in the body, their effect on the koshas, the organs they touch, as well as the doshas—when deciding which lines to work.

According to Ayurveda, certain organs are more closely linked with particular doshas. In identifying which dosha you want to work on in the massage, choosing sen lines that are also linked to that organ allows you to use sen lines and Ayurveda together. For example, Sen Ulangka and Lawusang run through the chest and lungs, and the chest is also related to the *kapha* dosha, so in a kapha-reducing massage you might choose to use these sen lines for greater effect.

Another deciding factor in choosing which sen line to use is the physical running of the line. If a client tells you he has a sore arm running from the side of the neck down toward the thumb, use Sen Thawari and Sahatsarangsi as part of the treatment in your massage.

Finally, you may want to work on a particular kosha as part of your massage, and certain energy lines penetrate deeper into the kosha bodies. Sen Sumana, for example, which runs along the primary chakra line, is a deep line that primarily touches the Wisdom and Blissful bodies.

As Lotus Palm students progress with Thai Yoga Massage pathology treatments, they are encouraged to start the massage wherever it is most effective for that particular situation. The primary aspect that determines your massage and the sen lines you choose is the present moment and the needs of your client. Ask yourself:

- Is there a condition in the physical body that needs attention? If that is your focus, choose the appropriate sen line(s).
- Is balancing a dosha a more effective approach in this case? If so, choose the sen lines that work with that dosha.
- Is there a kosha on which you'd like to focus? Select the appropriate sen line for that kosha.
- If you want to work on two or three of these aspects at the same time, choose sen lines that also overlap. However, to begin with, keep it simple. It is better to have one clear-minded focus and explore it deeply rather than having your attention drawn all over the place at a surface level.

---

*For further explanation of the Ayurvedic doshas, please refer to the author's earlier text, *Thai Yoga Therapy for Your Body Type: An Ayurvedic Tradition.*

Finding the Sen Lines

Don't expect to feel a line of energy, a pulsation in your hand, or any such experience when you touch a sen line. This is the beginning of marginalization and also puts undue pressure on you if you don't feel it, as if you don't belong to the club or you're not sensitive enough. It doesn't really matter. From the thousands of students we have taught I can say with full confidence that all you need to do is put your heart into it and trust you are there, and let the universe take care of the rest. We are all born with the gift of touch.

There is also no best place or designated beginning point to a sen line, because the energy lines run in a circular motion. Although Lotus Palm often starts with the recipient in a sitting position, we honor everyone's individual approach.

EXPLORING THE SEN LINES

The following sections include traditional line drawings of the sen lines. The sen lines drawn and photographed on a live person are also provided in the color insert, where they have been somewhat simplified for easier comprehension. This chapter describes some of the important properties of each line and how to relate sen lines to the Ayurvedic doshas and the koshas.

In describing the path of the sen lines on the physical body I have mostly used everyday terms, and only in certain places do I refer to anatomical locations. This might seem cumbersome for some, but I decided on this approach to unite the traditional with the modern and to make the descriptions accessible for all.

Our school uses a series of landmarks to help students differentiate the sen lines and make them easier to follow. Whether working on paper or on a partner, begin by identifying the bodily landmarks described below—and shown on the photographs in the color insert—and connect the sen lines through the appropriate landmarks.

When massaging the sen lines, it's important to always respect the recipient in all ways—physically, ethically, and with common sense. Therefore, always abide by the universal ethics of propriety and do not touch anywhere close to the breast, genitals, or anus. Furthermore, you should always check in with regard to pressure and keep a regular eye on your partner. If you feel the body tense, or receive visual cues from the eyes squinting or the face grimacing, reduce your pressure.

There are many techniques for working the lines, using the hands, thumbs, forearms, knees, and feet. Additionally, there are many different hand techniques, some in which the thumbs are right next to each other, others when they are apart, and so on. The specific touch technique you choose to use will depend on the part of the body you're addressing and optimal body mechanics. The recipient's feet, legs, torso, back, head, and arms should all be considered separately and always conform to the four basics. Choose a stance that helps you to face your work, add the rhythmic rock that complements the stance, and choose an intelligent touch technique that allows for minimum effort and maximum results. Massaging the sen lines is a dancing meditation, like a pendulum that swings from side to side, and when you work from a place of comfort, you should feel the metta touch shine through to your recipient.

❁ SEN KALATHARI

Sen Kalathari is commonly referred to as the emotional line of the body. It runs concurrently with the principal arteries and, when worked on, acts as a second pump to the heart. In the Lotus Palm tradition, Sen Kalathari is used as the primary line in many treatments, as it covers the entire physical body as well as the five kosha bodies. It is also tridoshic, in that it can be used to help circulate energy that is beneficial to vata and kapha body types and also relaxes the highly charged pitta body type.

Treatment Properties

Sen Kalathari can be used in treating symptoms related to allergies, arthritis, asthma, calf muscle cramps, digestion, hernia, recovering from heart attack and stroke, knee pain, menstrual cramps, stiff neck, numbness of limbs and extremities, sciatica, sinusitis, varicose veins, epilepsy, and mental disorders.

Linking Organs, Sen Lines, Ayurveda, and Kosha

The organs are the way to link the sen lines with the dosha of Ayurveda. For example, Sen Kalathari goes through all of the vital organs, including the small intestine, a pitta organ; large intestine, a vata organ; and lungs, a kapha organ. Because it covers the whole body, it is considered tridoshic and can be used for all body types. Use Sen Kalathari when you want to give a pitta-reducing, vata-reducing, or kapha-reducing massage.*

SEN KALATHARI		
Primary Organs	**Doshas**	**Koshas**
Small intestine, large intestine, liver, spleen, stomach	Tridoshic	Primarily the mind-body, also touches all five koshas

Tracing the Inside Line
Foot

On the sole of the foot, use the image of a rising sun along the top of the heel with the rays shining out toward the five toes.

---

*While it may seem counterintuitive that what reduces vata can also reduce kapha, the result can be influenced by the intensity, pace, and specific postures chosen to stimulate the lines.

LANDMARK

+ Top round of the heel

Legs

From the top of the heel, continue in a straight line up the inside of the leg along the center of the calf muscle and adductor muscle.

LANDMARKS

+ Deep soft spot between the malleolus (bony protuberance on the side of the ankle) and Achilles tendon.
+ Top of the tibia bone just below the knee. Locate it by tracing the tibia bone, which curves at the knee, and finding the soft spot at the bottom of the curve.
+ Soft spot just beyond the knee. Locate it by cupping the knee and pointing your thumb at a 45° angle.

Note: Do not apply pressure on the knee and avoid coming close to the genital area.

Torso

From the leg, skip the groin area, find the center of the hip bone and draw a diagonal line that crosses at the navel, continuing through the nipples, and reaching the armpits.

LANDMARK

+ Center of hip

Note: Do not touch nipples or breasts.

Arms and Hands

From the armpit, continue in a straight line along the inside of the arm in the groove between the bicep and triceps.

From the crook of the elbow, move along the center of the forearm to the center of the wrist. Finish with five sun rays toward the fingertips.

LANDMARKS

+ Center of elbow
+ Center of wrist

Head

From the protruding angle of the collarbone, continue in a straight line up the neck, face, and head in line with the outer edge of the eye.

LANDMARK

♦ Protruding angle of the collarbone

Note: To join Sen Kalathari of the head with Sen Kalathari at the chest, draw a line from the protruding angle of the collarbone toward the armpit.

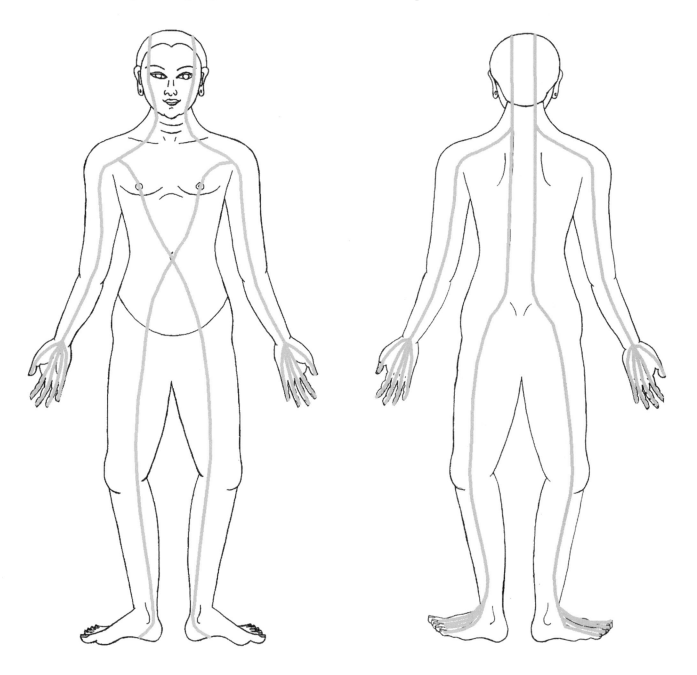

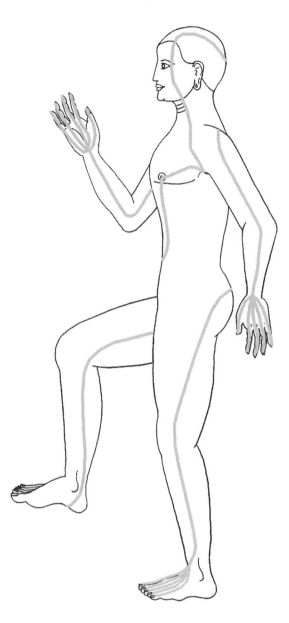

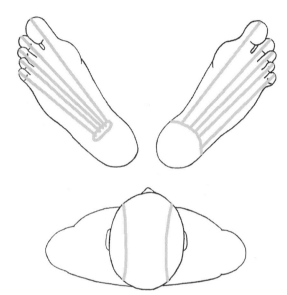

Tracing the Outside Line

Foot

On the top of the foot, from Gulpha marma (soft spot between the ankle bones),* continue with five sun rays to the toes.

LANDMARK
♦ Gulpha marma

---

*See page 52 for more information about the marmas.

Legs

From Gulpha marma, continue above the malleolus and in a straight line along the center of the leg, following the center of the calf muscle and the iliotibial (IT) band—the thick, fibrous tissue that runs along the outside of the leg—to the center of the hip bone.

LANDMARKS

- Spongy tendon between the Gulpha marma and the malleolus.
- Top of the tibia bone just before the knee. Locate it by tracing the tibia bone, which curves at the knee, and finding the soft spot at the bottom of the curve.
- On top of the IT band starting just beyond the knee. Locate it by cupping the knee and pointing your thumb at a 45° angle.

Note: Do not apply pressure on the knee, and keep your fingers in a fist when coming close to the hip bone so as to avoid the genital area.

Back and Head

From the hip bone, circle around the buttocks and curve in a sideways S until you reach the soft spot at the outer edge of the sacrum.

Continue in a straight line along the top of the paravertebral muscles on either side of the spine, staying close to the spine and neck, over the back and top of the head, coming around to meet the inside line at the outside edge of the eyes.

LANDMARK

- Soft spot at the outer edge of the sacrum

Note: We often refer to the top of the paravertebral muscles as "the hilltops." There is also "the valley" between the muscle and spine, which is the location of a different line.

Arms and Hands

From the paravertebral muscles, branch off under the ridge of the scapula making a straight line to the armpit.

Continue in a straight line along the center of the triceps and forearm until the middle of the wrist. Finish with five sun rays toward the fingertips.

LANDMARKS

- Where the ridge of the scapula meets the arm
- The center of the wrist

❈ SEN ITTHA AND SEN PINGKHALA

Sen Ittha (left side of body) and Sen Pingkhala (right side of body) are commonly referred to as the moon and sun lines, or the energy lines that help to balance the left and right sides of the body. Since they run along the back of the legs and close to the spine, they are particularly effective for people with back issues, one of the most common occurrences in people seeking relief from Thai Yoga Massage.

Treatment Properties

Sen Ittha and Sen Pingkhala can be used when treating symptoms related to arthritis, back pain, circulation issues, common cold, cough, eye pain, throat ache, abdominal issues, urinary tract issues, dizziness, diabetes, headaches, knee pain, menstrual cramps, stiff neck, and varicose veins.

Linking Organs, Sen Lines, Ayurveda, and Kosha

The organs are the way to link the sen lines with the dosha of Ayurveda. For example, Sen Ittha and Pingkhala go through the large intestine, which is a vata organ; and the lungs, a kapha organ. Use Sen Ittha and Pingkhala when you want to give a vata- or kapha-reducing massage.

SEN ITTHA, SEN PINGKHALA		
Primary Organs	**Doshas**	**Koshas**
Large intestine, lungs	Kapha, vata	Energy body, mind body

Tracing the Inside Line

Torso

Find the center of the hip bone and move in a straight line along the side of the sternum toward the inner edge of the collar bone.

LANDMARK
- ◆ Center of hip

Note: Do not touch the nipples or breasts.

Arms and Hands

Draw a straight line from armpit to armpit. From the armpit the line runs along the inside edge of the arm, along the edge of the bicep, turning in slightly at the elbow and continuing along the edge of the forearm up the side of the hand and the pinkie finger.

LANDMARKS

♦ Inner crook of elbow
♦ Side of wrist

Head

From the inner edge of the collarbone, continue in a straight line up the neck, past the corner of the lips, to the outer edge of the nostrils and inner edge of the eye.

LANDMARK

♦ None

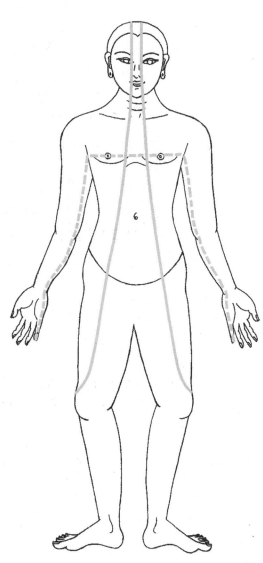
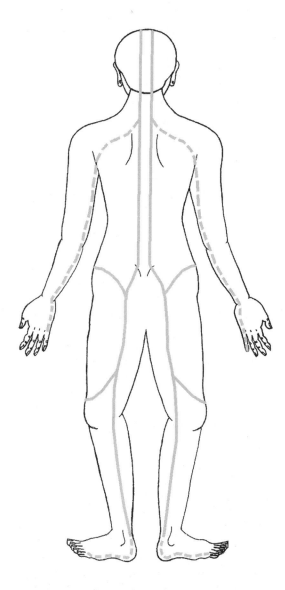

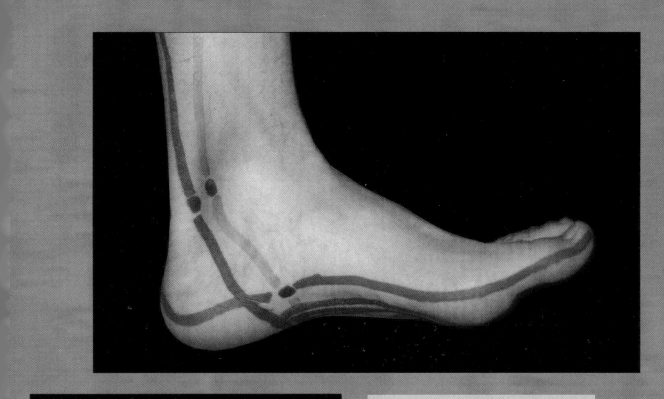

Sole of the foot

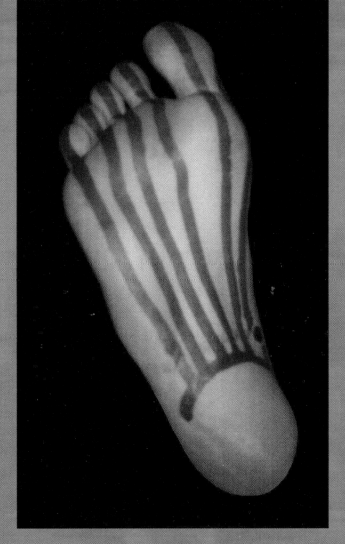

THE SEN LINES BROUGHT TO LIFE

Legend

- ◆ Red: Sen Kalathari
- ◆ Blue: Sen Ittha/Pingkhala
- ◆ Green: Sen Thawari/Sahatsarangsi
- ◆ Orange: Sen Sumana
- ◆ Purple: Sen Lawusang/Ulangka
- ◆ Brown: Sen Nanthakrawat/Khitchanna

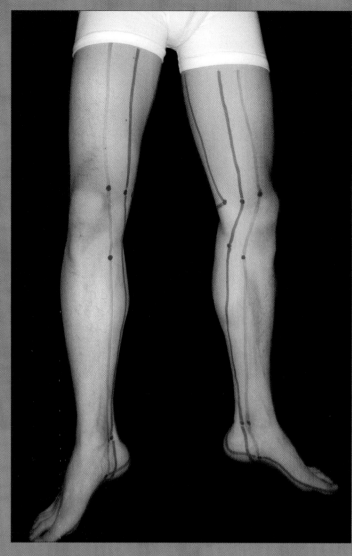

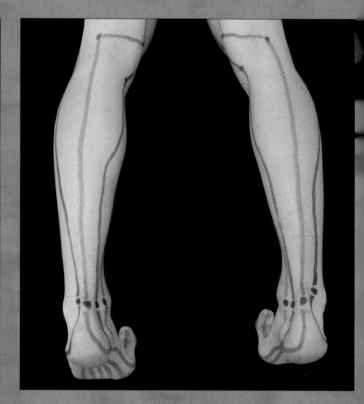

Inner leg

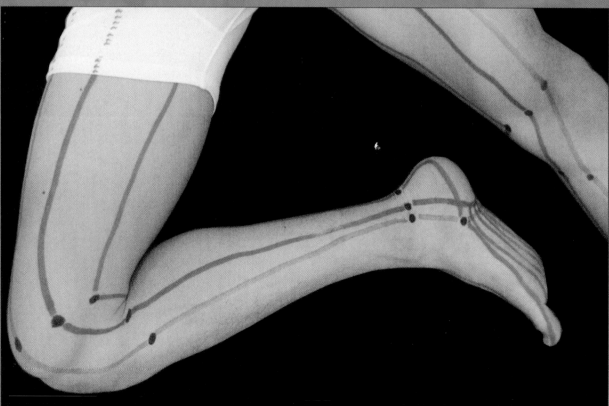

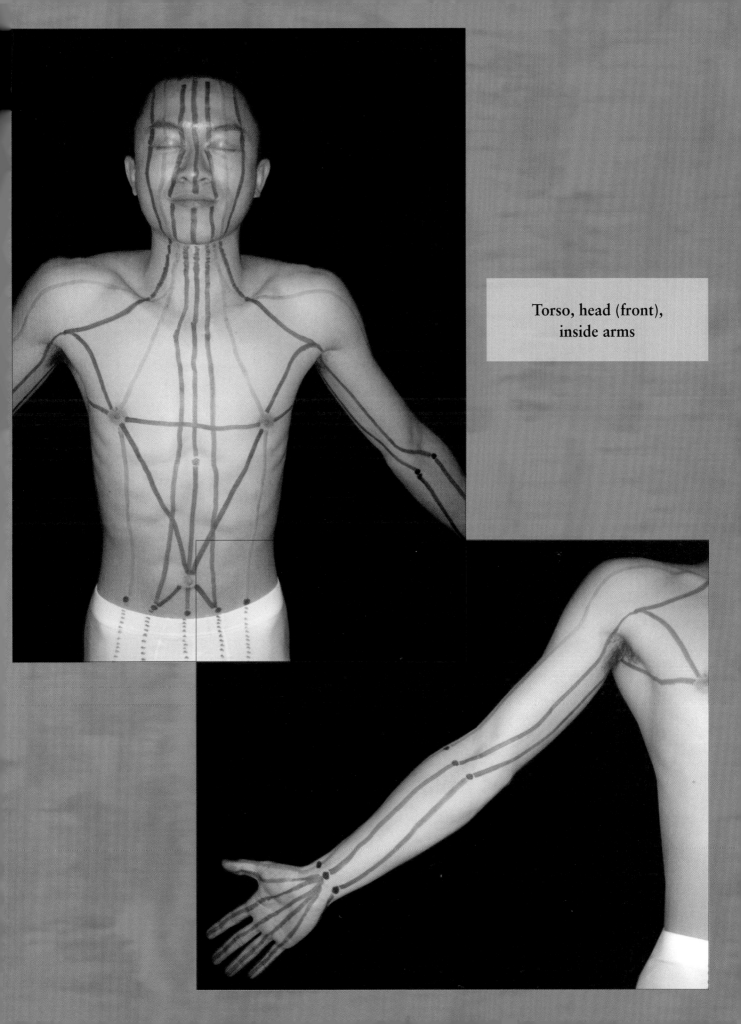

Torso, head (front),
inside arms

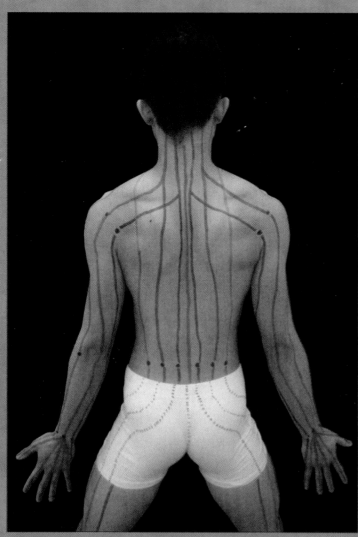

Upper back, back of shoulder, arms

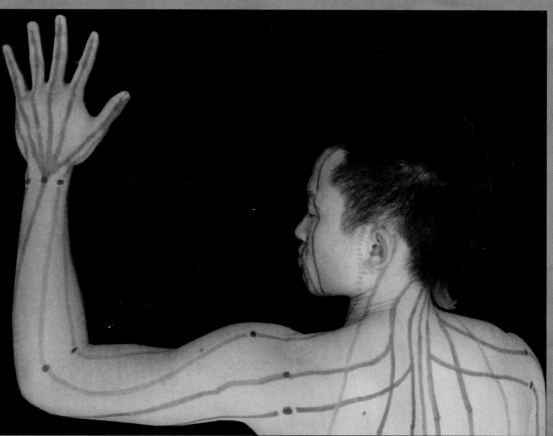

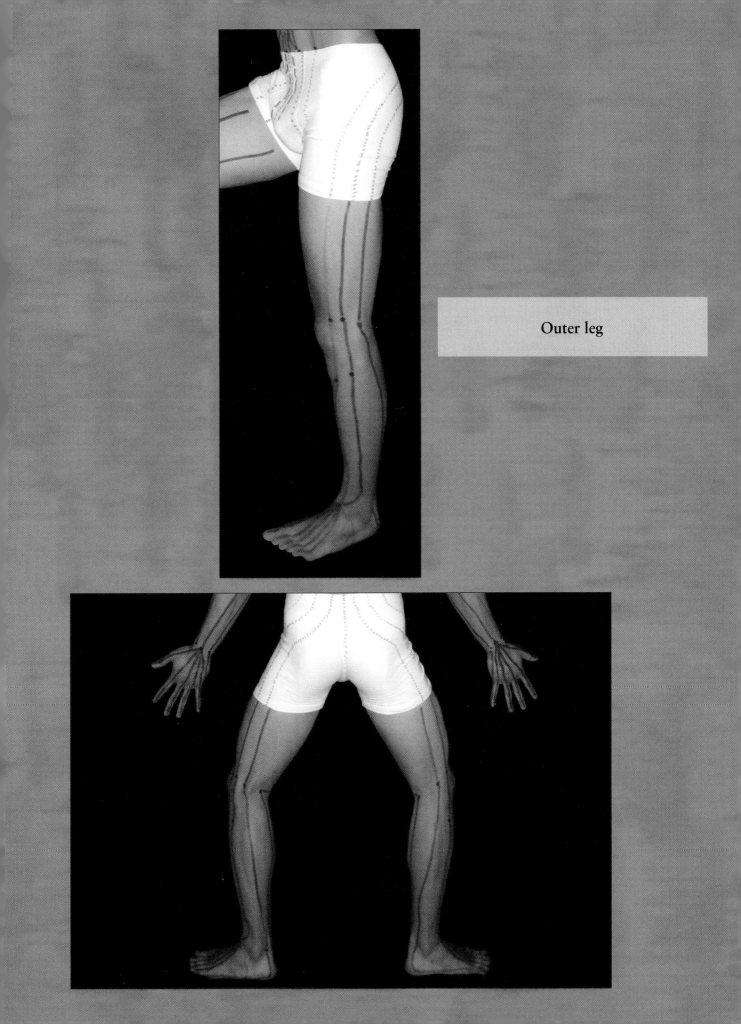

Outer leg

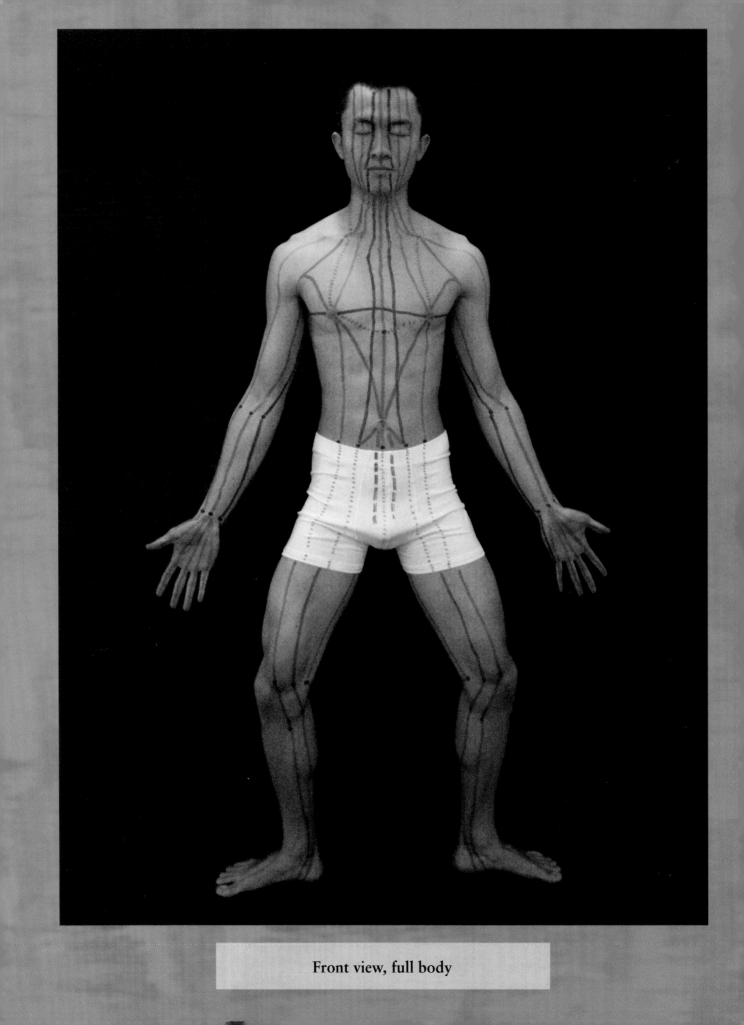

Front view, full body

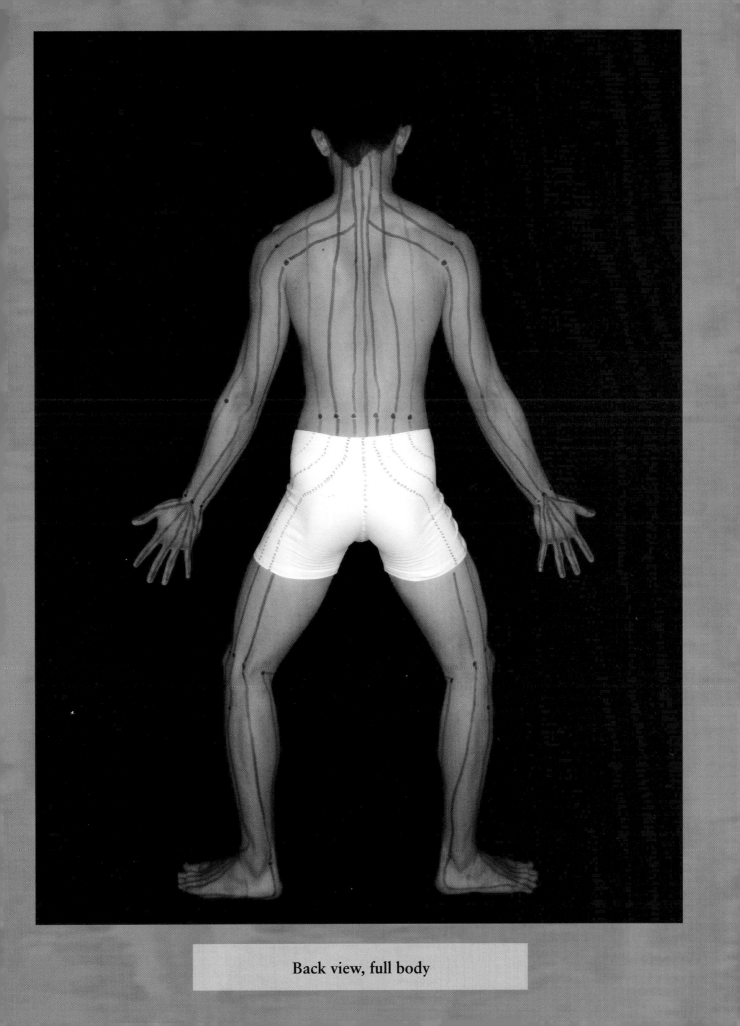

Back view, full body

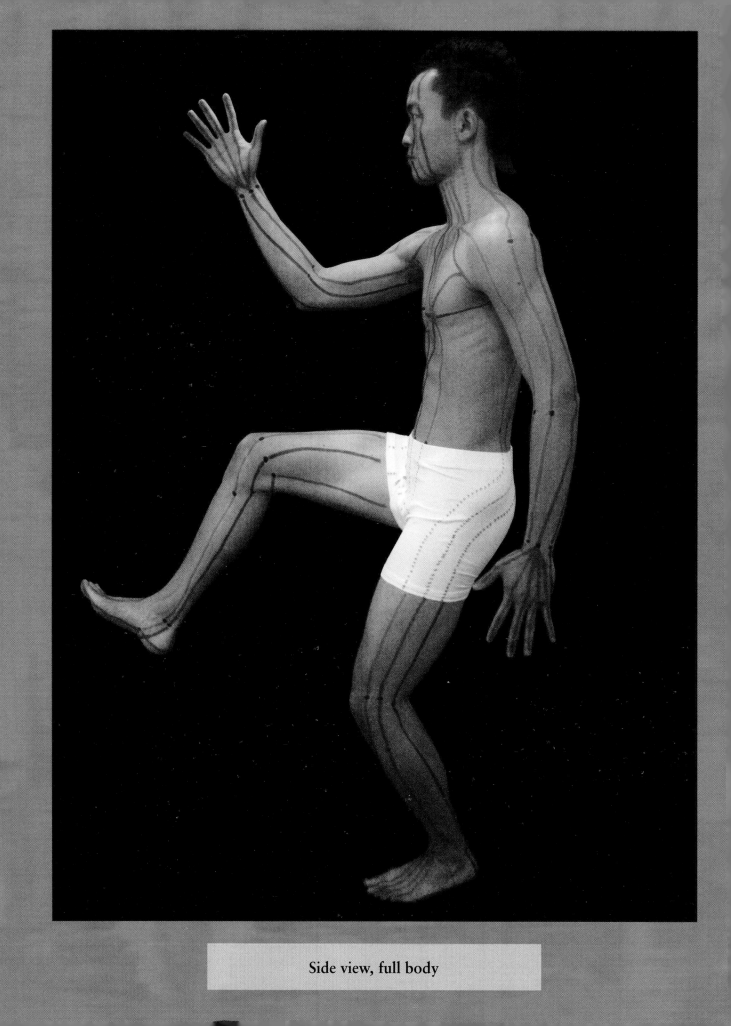

Side view, full body

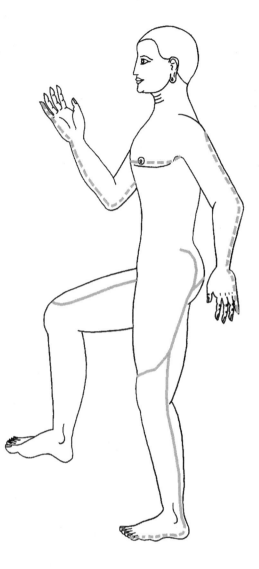

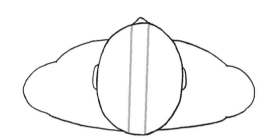

Tracing the Outside Line

Foot

Start from the outside edge of the pinkie toe, go along the outside of the foot, and travel around the heel.

LANDMARK
♦ None

Legs

From the outer edge of the heel, continue in a straight line above the Achilles tendon along the outside of the calf muscle and the outside of the quad muscle until the bottom of the hip bone.

LANDMARKS

♦ Soft spot just above the Achilles tendon

♦ Edge of the fibula

♦ "Guitar string tendon" just beyond the outer edge of the knee, found by bending the knee

Note: It is okay to press along the knee as long as you do not press on any bones.

Back

From the bottom of the hip bone, circle around the buttocks curving in a sideways S running parallel to Sen Kalathari until you reach the soft spot at the inner edge of the sacrum close to the spine.

Continue in a straight line along the valley between the paravertebral muscles and the spine all the way up to the neck, the back of the head, over the top, and meeting the inside line at the inside edge of the eyes.

LANDMARK

♦ Soft spot at the inner edge of the sacrum

Arms and Hands

From the paravertebral muscles, branch off at the center of scapula in a straight line to the armpit.

Continue in a straight line along the edge of the triceps and forearm until the back of the pinkie finger.

LANDMARK

♦ Where the side of the armpit meets the back. Locate this landmark first in order to identify where the line branches away from the valley next to the spine.

❁ SEN THAWARI AND SEN SAHATSARANGSI

Sen Thawari (right side of body) and Sahatsarangsi (left side of body) are connected to the vision and the eyes. Thawari literally means "origin at the right eye," and Sahatsarangsi means "origin at the left eye." Taken further, we can take this to mean a good workout of these lines can help with having deeper insight into the mind and wisdom bodies.

Treatment Properties

Sen Thawari and Sen Sahatsarangsi can be used when treating symptoms related to arthritis, high blood pressure, shoulder pain and frozen shoulder, varicose veins, facial paralysis, toothache, eye swelling, gastrointestinal diseases, knee pain, hernia, jaundice, depression, and numbness of legs, arms, and fingers.

Linking Organs, Sen Lines, Ayurveda, and Kosha

The organs are the way to link the sen lines with the dosha of Ayurveda. For example, Sen Thawari and Sahatsarangsi go through the large intestine, which is a vata organ. Use Sen Thawari and Sahatsarangsi when you want to give a vata-reducing massage.

SEN THAWARI, SEN SAHATSARANGSI		
Primary Organs	**Dosha**	**Koshas**
Large intestine, kidneys	Vata	Mind body, intellect body

Tracing the Inside Line

Foot

On the sole, just before the heel begins, make a horizontal straight line across the foot.

LANDMARK

- Soft spot on the instep of the foot, one thumbprint above the top of the heel

Legs

From the instep, continue in a straight line along the side of the foot just under the malleolus, and trace the muscle the entire length of the tibia as well as the inside edge of the quadriceps muscle.

LANDMARKS
- Soft spot just beside the malleolus
- Top of the tibia bone just before the knee. Locate it by tracing the tibia bone, which curves at the knee, and finding the soft spot at the top of the curve.
- Soft spot on the inside edge of the quadriceps just beyond the knee. Locate it by cupping the knee and pointing your thumb straight toward the shoulder.

Note: Do not apply pressure on the knee and avoid coming close to the genital area.

Torso

From the leg, skip the groin area; find the outside edge of the hip bone.

Make a straight line to the nipple and then turn inward 45° toward the center of the collar bone.

LANDMARK
- Outer edge of hip

Do not touch the nipples or breasts.

Arms and Hands

From the center of the collarbone, continue in a straight line toward the outer edge of the shoulder.

Move down the outer edge of the biceps and forearm, finishing at the tip of the thumb.

LANDMARKS
- Outside edge of elbow
- Soft spot on outside of wrist

Head

From the center of the collarbone, continue in a straight line up the neck, face, and head in line with the center of the eye.

LANDMARK
- None

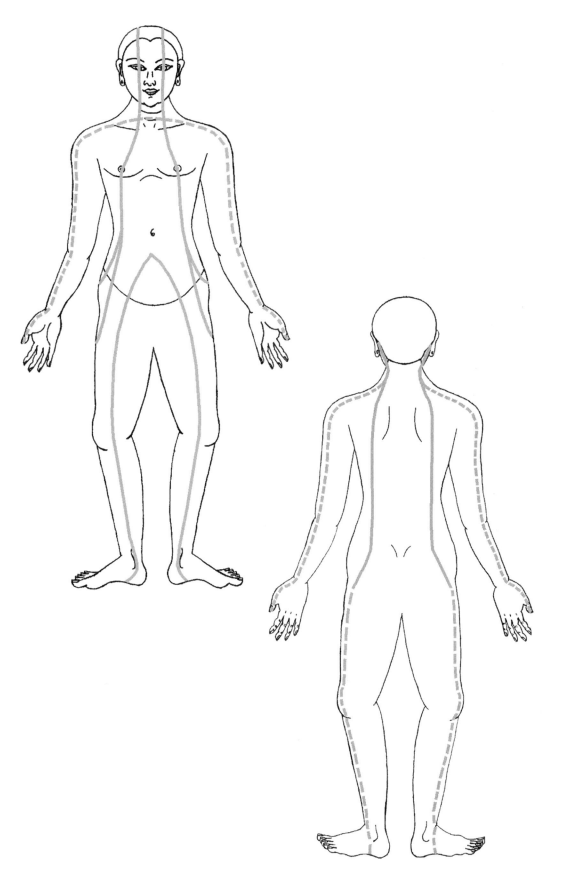

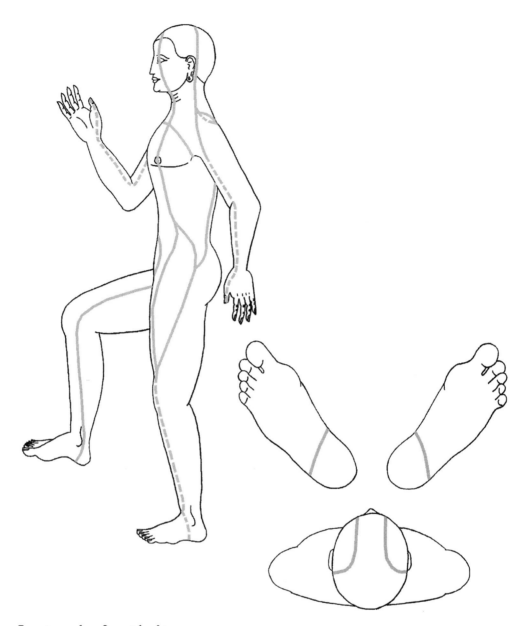

Tracing the Outside Line

Foot

From the blade of the foot one thumbprint above the heel, continue along the outside of the foot toward Gulpha marma.

LANDMARK
- Gulpha marma

Legs

From Gulpha marma continue in a straight line and trace the muscle just beside the tibia, as well as the outside edge of the quadriceps muscle until you reach the hip bone.

LANDMARKS
- Gulpha marma
- Top of the tibia bone just before the knee. Locate it by tracing the tibia bone, which curves at the knee, and finding the soft spot at the top of the curve.
- Soft spot on the outer edge of the quadriceps starting just beyond the knee. Locate it by cupping the knee and pointing your thumb straight toward the shoulder.

Note: Do not apply pressure on the knee, and keep your fingers in a fist when coming close to the hip bone so as to avoid the genital area.

Back and Head

From the hip bone, make a sharp circle around the buttocks in a sideways S, parallel to Sen Kalathari, until you reach the soft spot on the back of the pelvis, which is also in line with the lowest point of the scapula.

Continue along the outside of the back and over the scapula, the side of the neck, around the back of the ear, coming up to the top of the head, turning to come down the head and forehead to meet the inside line at the center of the eye.

LANDMARK
- Soft spot on the pelvis in line with the lowest point of the scapula

Arms and Hands

Branch off from the back along the trapezius muscle at the top of the shoulder.

Move from the bone at the edge of the shoulder (acromion process, or simply acromion) and continue in a straight line along the outside edge of the arm until you reach the tip of the thumb.

LANDMARK
- The acromion process

SEN SUMANA

Sen Sumana runs along the center of the spine and through the seven major chakras. It is similar to Sushumna nadi in yoga, in that it is a deep line activated by kundalini energy. Kundalini is said to be the dormant spiritual energy curled at the base of the spine, and when unleashed, it spirals up through the chakras, spinal column, and brain. With this unleashing comes an outpouring of vital energy and interconnectedness with the divine present moment. The line is connected with the mouth and its literal translation is "origin at the tongue."

Treatment Properties

Sen Sumana can be used when treating symptoms related to asthma, back pain, bronchitis, calf muscle cramps, circulation, heart disease, numbness of the legs, shoulder pain and frozen shoulder, sinus, digestion, abdominal pain, and common cold and cough.

Linking Organs, Sen Lines, Ayurveda, and Kosha

The organs are the way to link the sen lines with the dosha of Ayurveda. For example, Sen Sumana goes through the large intestine, which is a vata organ; the small intestine, which is a pitta organ; and the lungs, which are a kapha organ. Use Sen Sumana when you want to give a vata-, pitta-, or kapha-reducing massage.

SEN SUMANA

Primary Organs	Doshas	Kosha
Small intestine, large intestine, reproductive organs, lungs, heart	Tridoshic	Blissful body

Tracing the Line

Foot

Moves from the side of the big toe along the instep and curves along to the back of the heel.

LANDMARK
- None

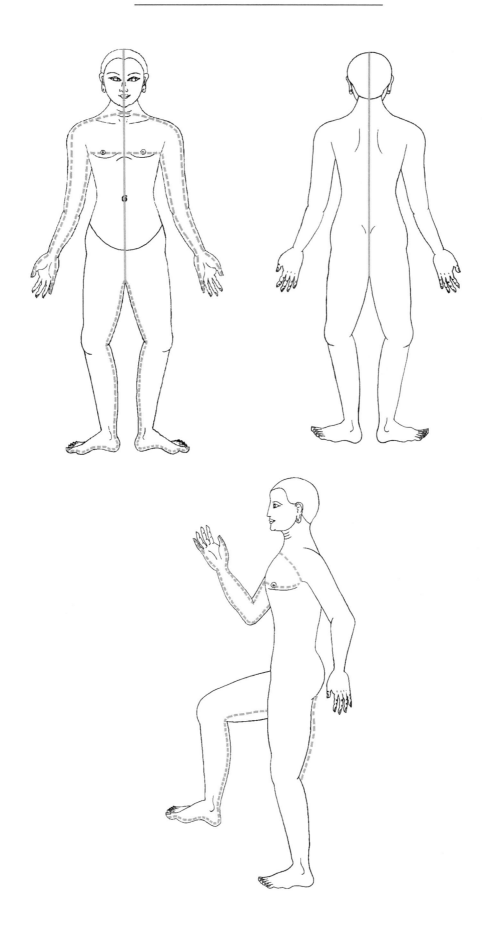

Legs

From the back of the heel, continue in a straight line up the Achilles tendon, along the back of the calf muscle until you reach the center of the knee.

Make a 45° turn inward to the thick tendon on the bottom inside of the knee, moving along the edge of the hamstring muscle and coming to the perineum.

LANDMARKS
- ✦ The Achilles tendon
- ✦ The back of the knee
- ✦ The soft spot on the thick tendon just beyond the knee

Note: Do not apply pressure on the knee, and avoid coming close to the genital area.

Torso

From the inside of the leg it travels up the perineum, the groin area, and the center line of the body through the navel, sternum, and in between the collarbones.

LANDMARK
- ✦ Lower abdomen, two inches below the navel

Note: Bypass the genital area.

Head

From between the collarbone, continue in a straight line up the throat, center of the mouth, nose, and third eye between the eyebrows until reaching the crown of the head.

LANDMARK
- ✦ None

Note: Do not touch the throat.

Back

From the crown of the head, continue down the vertebrae of the neck and back, joining up with the front line at the perineum.

LANDMARK
- ✦ None

Note: Do not apply direct pressure on any bones. Sen Sumana on the back is activated by stretching the spine and neck.

SEN ULANGKA AND SEN LAWUSANG

Sen Ulangka (right side of body) and Sen Lawusang (left side of body) are called upon in therapeutic treatments having to do with the ears, chest, and face. They are great lines to use for stiff necks and are thus particularly useful with a great many clients. The alternate names of these lines are Sen Chanthaphusang and Sen Rucham, which are literally translated as "origin at the left ear" and "origin at the right ear."

Treatment Properties

Sen Ulangka and Sen Lawusang can be used when treating symptoms related to ear pain or infection, cough, chest pain, facial paralysis, toothache, gastrointestinal issues, and heartburn.

Linking Organs, Sen Lines, Ayurveda, and Kosha

The organs are the way to link the sen lines with the dosha of Ayurveda. For example, Sen Ulangka and Lawusang go through the ears, which are a vata organ; and the lungs, which are a kapha organ. Use Sen Ulangka and Lawusang when you want to give a vata- or kapha-reducing massage.

SEN ULANGKA, SEN LAWUSANG

Primary Organs	Doshas	Koshas
Ears, lungs	Vata, kapha	Energetic, mind-body

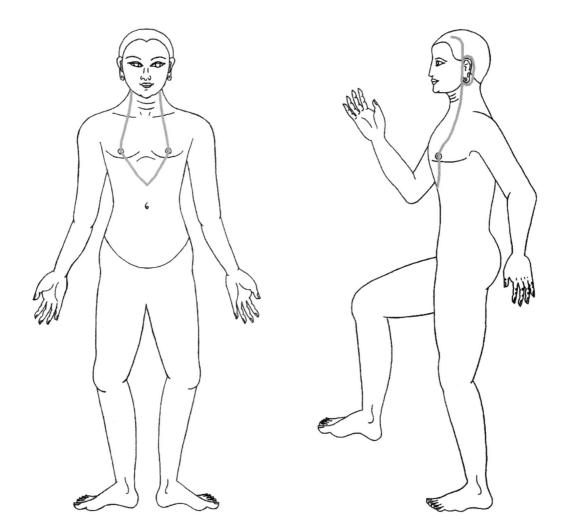

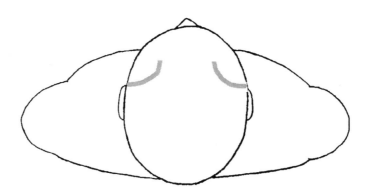

Tracing the Line

Torso

From the bottom of the sternum, make a 45° angle toward the nipples.

Move in a straight line from the nipples up the chest and the outside of the neck.

LANDMARK

♦ The bottom of the sternum

Note: Do not touch the nipples or breasts.

Head

From the side of the neck, continue along the side of the jaw, then branch off to make a complete circle of the ear.

Continue along the side of the face to the top of the head, angling forward and stopping in the center of the head, joining up with Sen Kalathari in line with the outer edge of the eye.

LANDMARK

♦ None

❧ SEN NANTHAKRAWAT AND SEN KHITCHANNA

Sen Nanthakrawat and Khitchanna are part of the traditional sip sen, or ten energy lines, but not that much is known about them and they are not often used in Thai Yoga Massage treatments. The lines run with the reproductive and waste-releasing organs; one runs along the pubic bone and the other runs right along the genital organs. You can access the lines only by massaging the abdomen.

Treatment Properties

Sen Nanthakrawat and Sen Khitchanna can be used when treating symptoms related to the urinary tract, infertility, impotence, irregular menstruation, diarrhea, and abdominal pain.

Linking Organs, Sen Lines, Ayurveda, and Kosha

The organs are the way to link the sen lines with the dosha of Ayurveda. For example, Sen Nanthakrawat and Khitchanna go through the reproductive and waste organs, which are vata organs. Use Sen Nanthakrawat and Khitchanna when you want to give a vata-reducing massage.

SEN NANTHAKRAWAT, SEN KHITCHANNA

Primary Organs	Dosha	Kosha
Reproductive, waste-releasing	Vata	Physical body

Tracing the Line

Torso

From the navel, moves in a straight line toward the perineum and anus.

LANDMARK
- Navel

Note: Massage only on the abdomen.

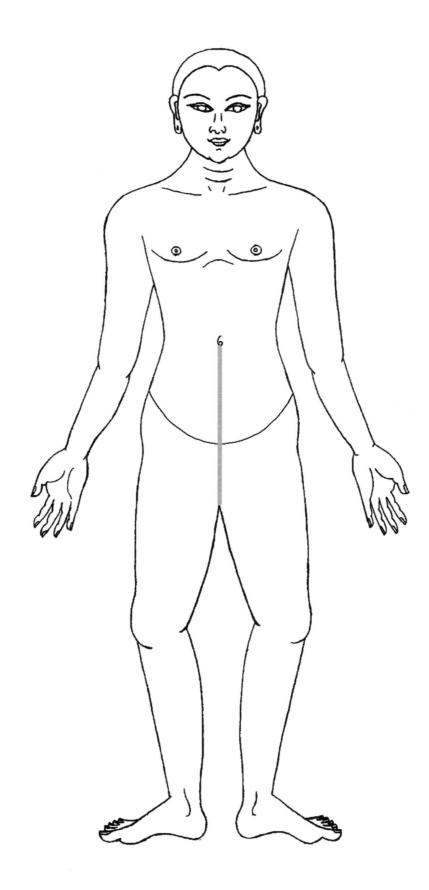

INTRODUCTION TO MARMA THERAPY

The Ayurvedic system includes 107 vital energy points, or marmas, that exist throughout the human body.* These points are important hubs of pranic energy that can be stimulated to increase energy flow, remove blockages, or even tap into hidden energy reserves.

The eighteen marmas selected here (see figure) are considered to be major points by virtue of their strong therapeutic values. Because of their size and location, these points are also among the easiest to work on within a Thai Yoga Massage format. Seven of the marma points presented here directly correspond to the seven chakras, the vital energy centers aligned along the spinal column. Stimulating these points during a massage session effectively releases a flow of energy throughout the entire chakra system.

Marmas are most easily stimulated by pressure applied with the thumb, the main pranic channel in the hand. However, the index finger, knuckle, heel of the hand, elbows, arms, knees, and feet can also be used with many of the marma points. The amount of recommended pressure varies according to the needs of your recipient.

Before beginning to apply marma pressure, bring your full awareness to the therapeutic properties and location of the specific marma point you will be addressing. Apply gentle pressure with your thumb and gradually pour your body weight into it.

Apply pressure for approximately five to ten seconds for general upkeep, or for up to one minute for deeper therapy. In order to prevent injury or discomfort, be sure to use the pad of the thumb. Direct pressure or circular motion can be applied, followed by a gentle massage of the region.

As you work on the marmas, visualize each point as an essential transfer station that sends a free and peaceful flow of energy throughout the region. Direct your own breathing to the marma point, inhaling positive healing energy and exhaling negativity and tension. You may also direct your recipient to breathe into a marma point that seems particularly tender or stagnant.

When experiencing marma pressure your client may feel a range of sensations—a delicious sense of release, a stimulation of energy, or a sense of lightness directly following the removal of pressure. If your client experiences pain, there may be a blockage or stagnant energy at that point. In such cases, work only as deep as your client is comfortable.

Never work on the marma points of a client who is pregnant, diagnosed with cancer, or suffering from inflammation or a skin disorder. Points on the face, head, and abdomen are more sensitive, so apply less pressure to these areas. Points on the arms, legs,

*This information was originally provided in *Thai Yoga Therapy for Your Body Type*. For a more in-depth discussion of marmas, please refer to that book.

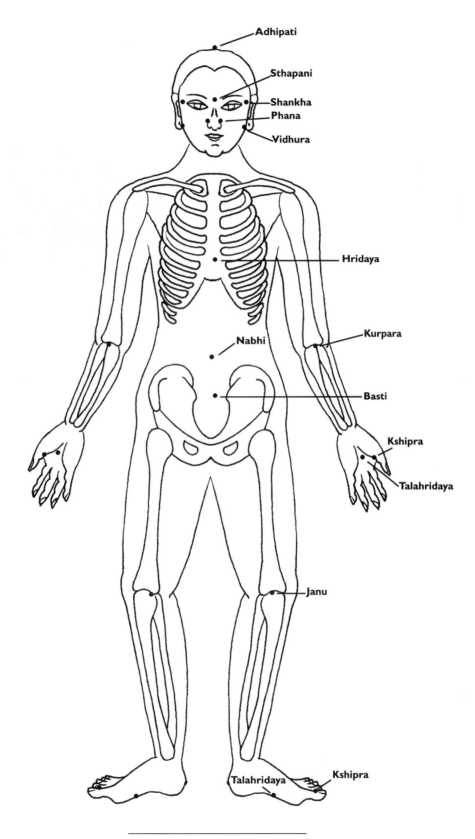

Key marma points: front view

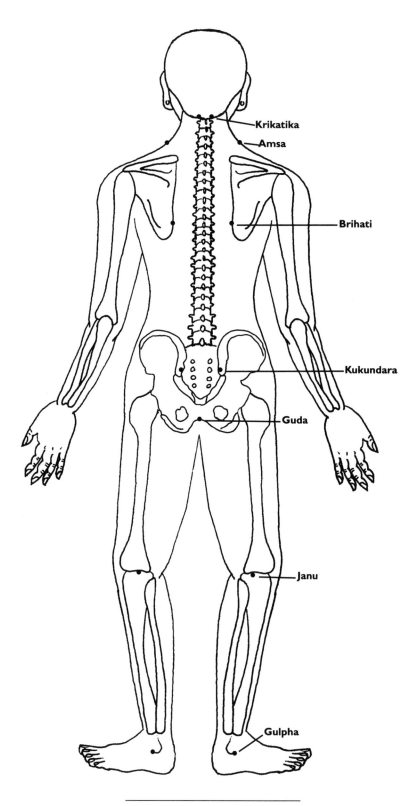

Key marma points: back view

feet, and hands are easiest to work on and can be very powerful in their effects.

In order to maintain the even distribution of energy, be sure to massage the marma points on both the right and left sides of the body. When working on marmas with multiple locations, such as the kshipra point located on the hands and feet, make sure to massage both the lower and upper points to prevent an imbalance of energy.

MASSAGE PATHWAYS QUESTION AND ANSWER

Working with the sen lines and marmas is both subtle and complex. This section will attempt to answer as many questions as possible regarding their use in Thai Yoga Massage.

Do the sen lines have a directional flow?

No. There is no directional flow but there is a general consensus among many of the schools that you start to work the energy lines from the feet and work your way up the body. At the start of your training, Lotus Palm chooses to work with the recipient sitting for several reasons:

- As with a yoga practice, when you start sitting you can end your massage in a supine position, lying face up in a state of deep relaxation. This allows the recipient to reap the most benefit from the practice, much like pressing the save button on your computer when you're finished with your work.
- If you start with the foot sequence you'll end with the recipient sitting, and it's much more difficult to prop up a restful body. Also, awakening that energy too abruptly doesn't lend itself to a yoga ending.
- When we spread out the work on the body we balance the session rather than overworking one half at a time. If you start with the feet and move up the legs, half the massage may be over before you even touch the upper part of the body.
- In the West, the primary areas of need and attention are often the shoulders and back. When you start with the recipient sitting you help her to let go and fully relax into the massage before continuing with the feet.

How do you know when a line is out of balance?

The practice of Thai Yoga Massage is generally practiced as a full-body, energetic workout, and we believe that any imbalance that occurs will be adjusted through this process. Since I do not promote or suggest knowing precisely what an energy line feels like, I must leave it to the practitioner to use the tools available, combined with your intuition. There are no precise measurements and I do not want to influence you.

What I would caution against is any judgment of a particular situation. It is extremely rare to find a walking Buddha in your midst, therefore everyone is out of balance and it is just a question of degree, so you should use the energy lines in some form for pretty much everyone.

How do you know if a line is blocked?
Does that happen, and if so, what do we do?

There is no such thing as an energy thermometer that measures where the current is flowing or not. It is not something that can be substantiated by numbers, so don't worry about that too much. Put your heart into the practice and use the physical application of metta toward your client. That's what counts. Your work is to massage the energy lines, to embody the principles of Ayurveda in your practice, to stretch, and to trust that any blockages will release at the client's own doing. You ensure you are practicing safely and respectfully by asking for feedback, especially when working with what is perceived as deep pressure.

What are the different ways to use
Thumb Chasing Thumb and Palm Chasing Palm?

In Thai Yoga Massage there are many different ways to work the energy lines, and two of the greatest are palming and thumbing. There are different ways and different schools of walking the lines with your thumbs and palm. They are all good. Find a way that is logical for your memory and your comfort so that you can dance and flow with the energy lines. For more specific details, the way to learn is to take a class.

Are there any other hand techniques beyond
palming and thumbing for working the energy lines?

There are many techniques to work the energy lines, specifically one called Thumb over Thumb Double Push. This technique is applied by using a first layer of pressure with your thumbs side by side and then following it by staying on the same spot and adding deeper pressure with your thumbs.

Can a massage tool be used to work the energy lines?

Yes indeed. The only issue is that your sensitivity will initially be reduced. Whenever you use tools you should continue to palpate through your tools and develop the sensitivity in the tools as an extension of your hand. Not only is this possible, it can make a big difference to your long-term practice.

What is the best posture to work the sen lines when the recipient is lying on her back with legs extended and you are working from the side?

You must always consider your own body. Make sure the recipient is lying in a position that is conducive not only to his relaxation but also to your working ease. It will help you to use props and good stances, and enable you to knee walk. Some of the key factors for good posture are to find the right distance, work so you do not hyperextend your wrist, and put no extraordinary stress on your body and thumbs. In other words, the four basics and the three gems we teach should be studied and utilized diligently, and always remember to see if you can do better with the next one. As I often say, the end of one journey is the beginning of the next; in this case, every massage is a learning experience that takes you to the next level.

Some of the sen lines cross the skeletal structure of the body. Is it okay to apply pressure there?

In general, applying reasonable pressure on certain boney areas, such as the sacrum, the dorsal of the foot, and the scapula can bring significant relief. However, there are places on the body that should be approached very cautiously, including the shin bone, the humerus, and the spinal area, especially the cervical spine, just to name a few.

Is it ever okay to press the knee?

In general, do not hyperextend the knee, put pressure on the patella, or torque the knees. However, there are sequences in which you do massage the knees. This has to be taught and applied with precautions, and it is best learned in the classroom.

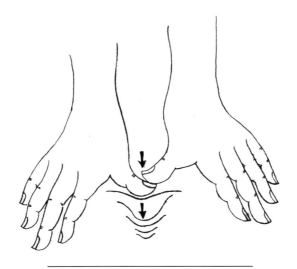

Thumb Over Thumb Double Push

What kind of pressure should be used when working the sen lines?

The rocking pressure of your body is generally best. It is a firm, stable, dancing pressure that comes from the leverage of using your body weight. But then again, there are places in the physical body that demand a stronger workout, where you may dig in to the body and sen lines. One such example is massaging the back. In this case be careful not to overuse your palms or thumbs, and be aware that repetitive strain is the most common injury to a practitioner. You should challenge yourself to use other parts of your body, including knees, elbows, and palms over thumb.

Is it better to work the energy lines directly on the skin?

Not necessarily. Thai Yoga Massage is just as effective through comfortable clothing. Wearing socks or not wearing socks is fine either way.

Do you need to work the sen lines harder on a muscular body and softer on a more narrow-framed body?

Yes, usually that is the case. It is through the physical that we go to the deeper layers. That is why in Thailand the massage is strong and deep. That is why we teach our students how to use their knees and feet as well as elbows and forearms to work the energy lines. It is to give everyone the freedom and flexibility to be light as a feather or strong as an ox, no matter what the situation dictates.

Can you hurt the client by overworking the sen lines?

On the physical level, yes; but energetically speaking, no. It could be compared to constantly wiping a window to keep it clear; you won't destroy it, but if you start to bang on the glass it might break.

It's important to work sensibly and strategically. You should assess the strengths and limitations of your client and see the massage as a slowly accelerating process. This is especially true for clients who have a lot of pain or seem out of shape.

How important is the breath, yours and the recipient's, when working the energy lines?

Practicing your massage mindfully includes being aware of your inhalation and exhalation and the natural rhythm of your breath. There are only certain times when working the sen lines during the massage that you coordinate your breath and the recipient's. Those times include working the back where you force out the breath, working the abdomen with a synchronized calming breath, and guiding the breath when putting a client into various stretches.

What happens if I work Sen Kalathari on the leg and don't get to it on the whole body?

Energetically, mindfully, spiritually you will touch the whole network. If it is not touched upon physically, that is okay. When you choose to work a particular line, do your best to work the entire line and keep your focus, but if you don't cover the line in its entirety, it's fine.

Should all of the ten sen lines be touched in a massage?

The way I was taught is that unless all the sen lines are worked on in a massage session, it shouldn't be called Thai Yoga Massage. Then again, the people who taught me sen lines didn't work all the lines during each session.

How do marma points relate to sen lines?

Marma points and sen lines are like subway lines with stations along the way, and some of them intersect. Some of them have more traffic activity and some have less. It is important to promote a free flow of energy so the stations and tunnels operate efficiently and everything is running smoothly. A logjam in one station will affect other stations along the route.

Are the landmarks on the sen lines marma points?

No. Please do not correlate them. The landmarks are basically a tangible guideline to help you map out the sen in the body.

Are the sen lines related to the chakras? Do the sen lines run along where the chakras are?

The seven major chakras run along Sen Sumana (Thai) or Sushumna nadi (Indian).

Does it make sense to start work on one side of the body for males and the other for females?

There are schools of thought that say to massage men starting on the right and women starting on the left, but in our school we don't use this distinction. We would rather you start in a familiar place. If anything at all, I prefer to start to work on the right side and end on the left, following the bowel direction.

How should the sen lines in the groin area be worked?

You should not work the sen lines in the groin area, even in your mind. It is not worth going into a controversial area that could jeopardize your practice, either physically or mentally. There have been millions of successful massages without touching that area.

How do the sen lines function in a broken or severed limb?

The energy body is contiguous, regardless of physical breaks or interruption. In a broken limb, address the sen line in the intact parts of the body and it will carry through the line. The energy body continues to exist in phantom limbs, and science has proven that people can continue to feel their limbs even when they are not there, so continue to work the sen lines as though the limbs were there.

If someone has a curved spine, are the sen lines also bent?

Energy is beyond physical appearance and body structure. When you start to follow the physical appearance, you are not working energy lines. Therefore, go with your feeling. It is not purely tactile. If you sense that the energy line moves in a straight line, then work it in that way and be careful not to compress the spine.

Can I apply oil on the sen line?

Traditionally oil is not used in Thai Yoga Massage.

Are certain energy lines stronger or more prominent in males versus females?

For the purposes of Thai Yoga Massage, no.

Can we use herbs or herbal compresses to activate the energy lines? What about a specific mantra?

People do use herbal compresses to work along the energy lines, and it is no less or more effective than using massage techniques. Mantras can be effective as well. Anything that gives you a reason to focus and a focal point can activate the line. Much of the effectiveness comes from your focused attention.

Does the color of the sen lines as drawn in this manual actually reflect the color of the line?

You can use these colors to direct your imagination and intention. I have reason to believe that the colors chosen by Asokananda and me have an intuitive connection to the sen lines.

Does it qualify as a Thai Yoga Massage if you do only directed sen line work?

There is a story of a seasoned yogini who was very flexible (as yoginis often are). No matter how much every Thai Yoga Massage therapist tried stretching her this way and that, she never really felt completely satisfied and relaxed. Then one day she received a massage in a small village in Thailand. The entire session was spent simply palming and thumbing, stimulating the sen lines throughout her body; no stretches, no postures, no fancy moves. This pure energy work and focus turned out to be the best massage of her life because the therapist was completely in tune and present, and this is what made the experience incredible.

The most important aspect of any massage is your focused attention. The rest takes care of itself, and it is good to let go of any preconception of what the massage is supposed to be so you can simply give the best massage possible. Some examples of situations in which you might practice only sen line work include people recovering from surgery, elderly people, anyone who cannot move the body too much, or someone you simply want to touch in a way that encourages stillness, meditation, and the inner journey.

Does it still qualify as a Thai Yoga Massage if you don't use the sen lines?

Metta is the one unifying energy that is present in all massages and makes all the difference in the world. When you use metta you touch the energy lines anyway, whether you are conscious of it or not.

Can working the energy lines release emotions?

Yes, and this seems especially prevalent in the West. When the energy lines are worked, there are past experiences buried deep in the various kosha bodies that are sometimes awakened. This can cause an emotional release that is totally fine and should be honored. By the same token, it's like eating a food you haven't had since your mother made it when you were young. It brings back strong emotional feelings that simply need to be felt and can then be released. You may start to have tears in your eyes, but it's not necessarily because you are sad, it may just be emotional energy—the interconnectedness, experience, and appreciation of life.

If you feel that a client is experiencing a deep release, it is recommended to stop the massage and focus on metta, giving the client the option to continue or not.

Can you use the sen lines to massage people with cancer or other serious illness?

This question has to be answered carefully and dealt with delicately. People who are suffering should not be deprived or marginalized from touch. Touch is usually much needed during this time. Serious illness comes in a thousand forms, so the best I can do here is give a general answer, and in such cases, always ask the doctor for permission. If the person gives full consent, then massage with a lot of care, attention, metta, and respect, and be aware not to overwork the sen lines. Use gentle to medium pressure on the sen lines without any strong pressure.

The opportunity to work on people who are suffering and provide some relief can be one of the most rewarding things in a massage therapist's career.

How many sen line massages can you receive in a week?

As many as you can afford with regard to both time and money. Your energy is like a window that you want to keep clear and flowing. You cannot clean it too many times. The more touch you receive, the better the quality of your life. People who really spend time on themselves are happier, and Thai Yoga Massage is one of the best things you can do to increase the quality of your life.

How many sen line massages can you give in a week?

It depends on how you practice. If you practice yoga, then you can perform a lot. However, if you do not practice yoga you will deplete your energy quickly. The four basics are what put you in the yoga practice. When you are stretching somebody's energy lines, make sure you are not pulling but that you are extending your own energy lines and stretching them as well. When you are doing a twist, make sure you have a stable stance or asana. Your breath should be controlled and focused. Last but not least, own your massage and make it fun, interesting, and beautiful. Use your passion to help others in their physical, energetic, and emotional balance.

Is there such a thing as negative energy, and if so, how do I protect myself against receiving it from a client?

Yes, indeed there is. If you sense trouble, please be aware of it and stay alert. Sometimes you can refuse a massage for that reason. If someone comes in with aggressive or sexual energy, keep yourself safe by excusing yourself with a ready-made diplomatic reason. If you feel as though someone is giving you negative energy, remember that the mind can supersede anything—it is that powerful. If you decide not to take the energy, it won't come to you, so you have to make a decision. That's the first thing you should do—declare you're not taking this energy. Block it out by having this self-defense. Afterward you can do a self-cleansing with any tradition familiar to you. Some people use sage, crystals, showering, or meditation. Most important of all is to remember that you have the ability to simply refuse it.

Can sen lines be massaged from a distance?

Yes, there is such a thing as distance Thai Yoga Massage transmission. In the spirit of yoga, the five kosha bodies of man are interconnected and we are all connected to a universal source. As such, there is a possibility of sending and directing wellness at a distance.

This is only a mere belief that might not hold much truth, but it is the power of manifestation. If you continue to believe and manifest the energy of the practice, it can turn into something tangible right in front of you. This is how you continue your growth, your interest, your skills, your business, and your practice of Thai Yoga Massage.

Can you massage your own energy lines?

Yes, you can massage your own energy lines with yoga poses, as well as through intentional touch. Self-massage in a meditative state—that is, not in front of the TV—is also a great way to deepen your sensitivity to the energy lines.

How many traditions are there for sen lines?

There are as many traditions as there are masters teaching it. The sen lines are closely related to the yoga nadis in language and source.

Do the northern and southern styles of Thai Yoga Massage have different approaches to working the energy lines?

The style from northern Thailand is slightly more dynamic in its approach: It emphasizes the techniques of palming and thumbing while using a gradual compression upon the energy lines. The southern style takes a more relaxed approach: It emphasizes the technique of plucking, in which the practitioner uses his fingers to strum or stimulate the nerves running along the energy lines. In the south they apply pressure and release with a pluck.

How accurate are the Lotus Palm sen lines?

Lotus Palm is accurate in its tradition and bodily landmarks. There is no standardization in the field, but the Lotus Palm energy-line tradition may be the most widespread. This is because Asokananda and I collaborated on a set of drawings that was published in Thailand, and most established massage schools display these charts as the standard for sen lines. Our worldwide influence has been circumstantial and was never intended.

With no unified standard for the drawing of the lines, it becomes very easy for anyone to develop drawings and call it their tradition, and then it seems cast in stone and unshakeable. From my perspective, we are in a place where today's art is tomorrow's tradition. I believe and hope that people understand that holding on to anything too strongly and seeing it as the only way is a big mistake. The Lotus Palm approach promotes simplicity, effectiveness, understanding, and an openness to interpretation, but when there are many masters, there are many approaches to working the sen lines.

What was your source of information in drawing the lines?

There were several sources: the epigraphs at Wat Po temple used by Asokananda in his first book, *The Art of Traditional Thai Massage,* which was the first published book on Thai Yoga Massage in a foreign language; we compared the yoga nadis with the Chinese meridians (jing luo); and most importantly, our own teaching experience and the teachings of Thai masters Chaiyuth and Pichet.

Your original drawings included many dotted lines. What are those and why don't they appear in the color insert photos?

During our days of research, Asokananda and I found that some parts of the lines run one on top of the other. With many years of practice I have found it very confusing to teach that aspect to people. Because those sections are also of lesser importance, we decided to simplify and take those parts of the lines out. It does not dilute the process.

Everything can be improved upon and that's what we have done. It is a newer model that is lighter, faster, and easier to use. When you keep something simple you make it universal, in that everyone has the ability to teach it, to learn it, and to benefit from it. That speaks directly to our philosophy of life and our goal of contributing to a better world.

Are the sen lines the theoretical foundation of Thai Yoga Massage?

This depends on whom you ask. For me it comes down to an understanding of the meaning of the word *theory*. I have long held that a theory is a set of principles that gives meaning to an art form.

Considering that there is no standardization and every teacher has his own use of the lines, understanding, and experience, the sen lines are certainly a theory that is based primarily on experience and is transmitted through deep intuition and long-term apprenticeship before one finally reaches mastery. Since these are lines that are difficult to learn academically and share universally, I call it an "open theory."

As for Lotus Palm, we decided to make Ayurveda central to our theoretical foundation for understanding how Thai Yoga Massage works and how to put it to best use. This comes back to an understanding of what makes for a strong theoretical foundation. Ayurveda has a long-established unified tradition that can be explained in principles that are easily transferable. With Ayurveda we can get the same results as with sen lines, but in much less time, with much more clarity, and with a wider research base to help back it all up.

In traditional Thai Massage, why do you spend so much time working the legs?

This depends on whose tradition you are referring to, as my experience is that masters work whichever part of the body is most in need. At the same time, there are many schools that either created or follow a tradition of working the legs first, because of the belief that this is the way energy flows in the body. I can relate to this, but at the same time I take the approach of listening and becoming intuitively aware of what the body needs. Address the body according to whichever part is screaming the loudest: Massage me, open me up, help me to feel good!

When I first started Lotus Palm I practiced mostly by starting out on the legs, but some of the most consistent feedback I heard from clients receiving massage for the first time was that there was not enough work done on the back. That is not to say they did not enjoy the massage; it is just that when it's done properly, it's like having a meal so satisfying that all the senses are complete.

That being said, at Lotus Palm we emphasize the back as much as the legs. Lotus Palm has managed to save some time by choosing Sen Kalathari as the main workout, whereas the so-called traditional way does most of the energy lines on the inside and outside of the legs and not as much on the top of the body. In those cases, for a sixty- or ninety-minute massage you tend to spend the majority of your time on the legs. From my own personal experience of receiving massage, if so much time is spent on the lower half before moving on to the top, I end up feeling agitated when my legs are relaxed and my upper body is not touched.

Why are there so many different energy-line systems out there? Who is correct?

There are different ways of getting there. It's like taking a trip from New York to Montreal. One is a more scenic way, others more direct, some take you along a river, and others through the mountains. Choose the direction that resonates with you. All will get you there in the end.

Are the sen lines all from yoga and India?

It is difficult to trace the origins of all the lines. There are schools that say the lines have been influenced by the Chinese meridians, yoga, and native Thai practices. This is a debate I will not get involved in as it leads to nowhere. It is clear that Ittha, Pingkhala, and Sumana have an origin in yoga; as for the rest, I cannot say for certain.

How do the lines relate to yoga?

In yoga the practice of activating the Ida, Pingala, and Sushumna nadis is a big part of the theoretical practice. In Thai Yoga Massage these three lines are apparent, identical, and cognate. Therefore, Thai Yoga Massage is a yoga practice.

Are the sen lines specific to Thai Yoga Massage?

For now, yes, but I believe that in the future, when science has a better understanding and the eventual ability to prove energy lines more substantially, we could use it for other purposes.

Can you dissect the body and see energy lines?

Not at the time this book is being written. Research on the existence of energy lines has been taking place since at least the 1950s. At this point there is no conclusive, widely accepted proof that shows the energy lines, but with the universal popularization of Eastern forms of bodywork, it is safe to say that more time, effort, and money will be spent in the coming years to continue the research.

Is there a system of measuring the thickness of the energy lines or the depth of the kosha bodies?

No. Since the energy lines have not been verified scientifically, obviously they cannot be measured or even discussed in tangible terms. The whole energy body and our relationships are multidimensional, and you are constantly using your energy body to send and receive information. For example, how often do you look up at just the right moment to see someone looking right at you? If a religious master such as the Dalai Lama comes to town, I can feel his energy. There is also communication over vast distances. We've all received phone calls at the precise moment we were thinking about the person. So with all that being said, you cannot measure it, but it is felt.

What evidence supports the existence of the sen lines?

You just have to trust that they are there, just as we trust that the core of human nature is love. Furthermore, an entire country (Thailand) has been practicing it for thousands of years, treating millions and millions of people. They all use sen lines as a theoretical base for treatments, with many positive results. This is one clear, albeit circumstantial, piece of evidence I can provide.

What is the relationship between sen lines and Western anatomy?

Historically, anatomy of the musculoskeletal system has never been required learning for a Thai Yoga Massage therapist. This is in part because of the understanding that any discomfort in the physical body is a result of something happening on a finer level. The sen lines run beyond the physical level and toward the more subtle inner working of the body. The sen lines are part of Eastern anatomy, which says you should learn the energy pathways of the body in order to have effective treatments in Thai Yoga Massage.

As Thai Yoga Massage has spread to the West and encountered the traditions of Western massage, it has encountered musculoskeletal anatomy as an important part of the theory of a safe and effective massage practice. It can only benefit a Thai Yoga Massage practitioner to have further understanding of how the body is affected through the massage. We offer ninety hours of Western anatomy training at Lotus Palm as part of our 420-hour massage therapist training program, and it has been very well received.

My recommendation is to learn as much as you can from all of these traditions so you continue to refine your touch, awareness, and knowledge. Most important is to keep improving and developing your art in whatever way you are drawn to do so, as it is all relevant. Conversely, I can safely say that none of the traditional Thai masters have much understanding of Western anatomy, yet they have practiced their art very successfully over thousands of years.

What is the future of sen lines?

I don't see that there is any way that sen lines can be standardized and agreed upon like the traditional Chinese meridians in the foreseeable future, as there are simply too many theories out there and no strong leadership to unify them. Moreover, there are many people who have a tradition in different art and massage forms who will encounter Thai Yoga Massage and add their own two cents. The sen lines will continue to evolve and new theories will be added. Some people will use Chinese tradition, others yoga and Ayurveda, others Reiki, and so on. So you can look at it and be confused, but if you look at it in an open manner of the more the merrier and nobody is wrong and all are right, it adds to the richness of the sen lines in Thai Yoga Massage.

How do I go deeper to learn the sen?

The sen lines are like the gopi chant. It's heartfelt more than physically felt, and everyone can become an expert. The only way to go deeper is to trust yourself and keep practicing. It requires a lifetime of experiential learning that is quite literally right at your fingertips.

Advanced Practice Series

While some postures demand more skill and experience to execute, there are no "advanced postures" in Thai Yoga Massage, only advanced *practice*. Advanced practice requires drawing on the whole spectrum of postures and techniques learned here and in my previous books to provide safe, thorough, targeted treatment.

A general advanced practice series is presented in this chapter. Some of the postures will be familiar, and some are new. In either case, it is useful to remember that when you palm or thumb the various parts of the body, you also connect with the sen lines. In addition, remember that the energy of the massage should be geared to the Ayurvedic body type of the recipient, so for a vata-dominant client, your movements will be soothing and gentle, for pitta they will be steady and relaxing, and for kapha, energetic and stimulating.

As you practice these postures, be mindful of maintaining one of the key stances. Also, when applying a technique, no matter how subtle, always bear in mind the rhythmic rocking dance methods of Bamboo, Forward, and Whirlpool Rock.

Always practice in a meditative mode to open up the heart; be aware and listen to the needs of your body as well as those of the recipient. Practice with peaceful, loving kindness, and have empathy for the being you are working with. This is the spirit of metta, which makes the healing more potent and meaningful.

Most important, always approach your work with ease, remembering what a privilege and joy it is to be able to help others and to physically express metta in motion.

❦ SITTING POSTURES

Westerners spend great amounts of time sitting in chairs and automobiles, which allows the bulk of our physical tension to accumulate in our heads and shoulders. Thus, a Lotus Palm Thai Yoga Massage generally begins by releasing and opening the upper body first.

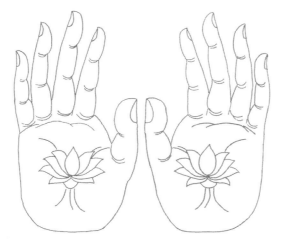

*Indicates postures taught in Lotus Palm's most advanced course, Thai Yoga Massage 6.

Namaskar

Namaskar is a traditional Hindu salutation, similar to Namaste, meaning that you are bowing to, or honoring, the Divine within the recipient.

The massage begins by standing at a comfortable distance from your client with legs shoulder-width apart, hands joined in a prayer position near the heart.

This is the moment to:

♦ Collect yourself and focus your awareness
♦ Prepare for the massage
♦ Become connected to the recipient
♦ Work with metta

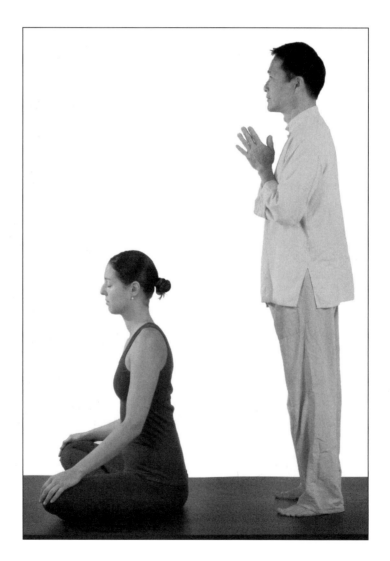

Palming Shoulders

- In the Tai Chi stance, support the back of the recipient.
- Keeping your back and arms straight, exhale your body weight onto your recipient's shoulders.
- Use a forward rock to palm the shoulders.
- The direction of pressure is straight down.

Precaution: Avoid pressing on the bones (clavicle and humerus), as this can be painful.

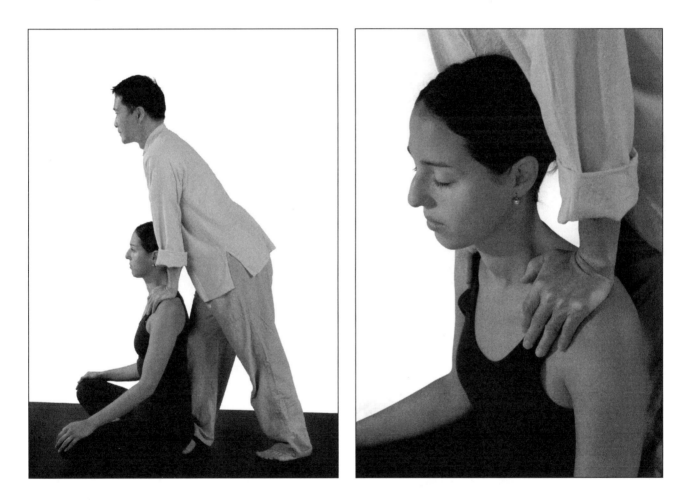

Splitting Rolling Pin

- ♦ Raise your right knee up in Warrior and gently tilt the recipient's head toward the right.
- ♦ Interlace your fingers and place your right forearm on the side of the head, left forearm or elbow on the shoulder.
- ♦ Sustain pressure with the right arm and roll out toward the edge of the shoulder with the left.
- ♦ Increase the stretch by gently extending both arms outward.
- ♦ Repeat on the other side.

Variation: You can also use your elbow to apply gradual pressure on the Amsa marma point located in the center of the trapezius, midway between the base of the neck and the edge of the shoulder. Place your left elbow on Amsa marma and gently sink in with gradual pressure. Hold for five to fifteen seconds.

Precaution: Make sure to keep contact on the muscles, avoiding any bones.

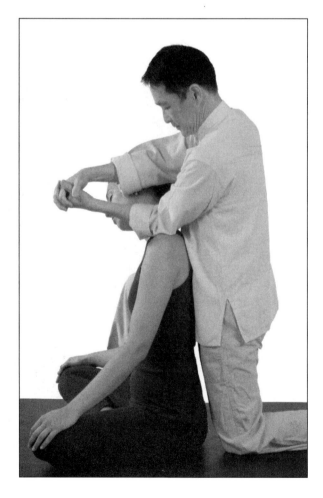 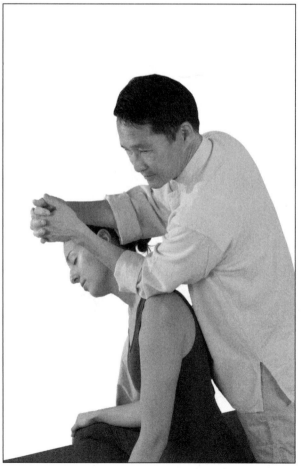

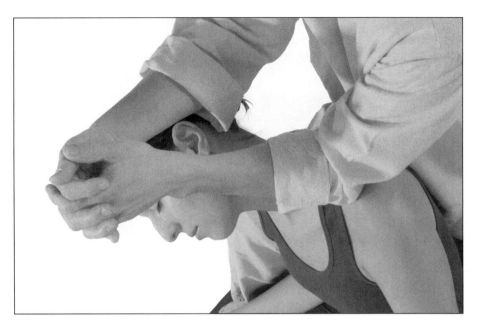

Ultimate Rolling Pin

- ◆ Bring your right knee in front of the recipient's thigh.
- ◆ Gently rest the recipient's head on your right thigh.
- ◆ Your right hand should be supporting the recipient's head while you use your left forearm or elbow to rock in and roll along the neck and toward the shoulder.
- ◆ You can comfortably reach Amsa marma from this position and also perform a neck massage.
- ◆ Gently bring the recipient's head to an upright position.
- ◆ Repeat on the other side.

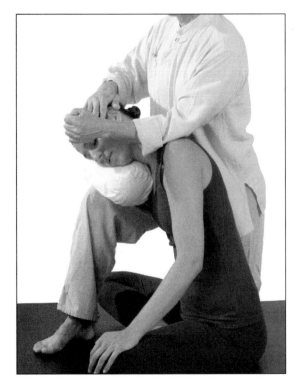

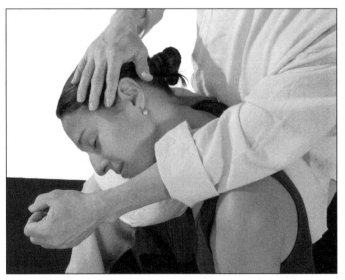

Double Water Pump

- ♦ In Kneeling Diamond stance, raise the recipient's arms and place the hands on the back of the head.
- ♦ Ask the recipient to interlace her fingers.
- ♦ Come into Open Archer stance, placing your right knee on the sacrum.
- ♦ Place your right elbow at the top of the shoulder and hold the recipient's hands.
- ♦ Use your left hand to support the head, pushing it forward.
- ♦ Elbow down the muscle between the scapula and spine.
- ♦ Change sides and stance to work on the left shoulder.

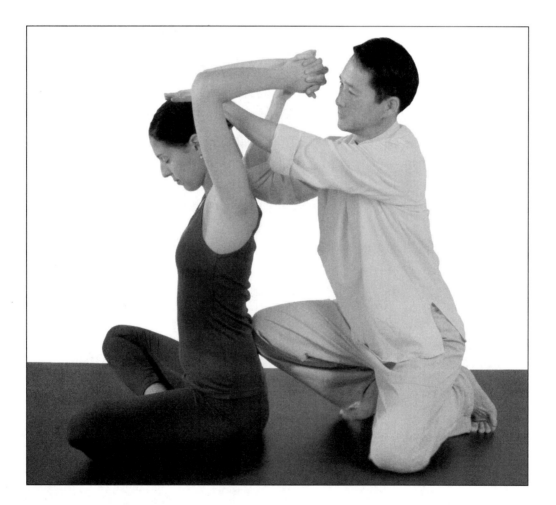

Metta Hug

- Sit in Open Diamond stance, remaining very close to your client, hugging her thighs with your legs. (Use a pillow if necessary.)
- Bring her hands behind her neck, interlacing her fingers and joining her elbows together in front.
- Interlace your fingers and hold her elbows.
- Gently lean back while pressing down on her elbows, pushing your chest into her back. (Women should place a thick cushion or folded blanket between themselves and the recipient to reduce contact with the breasts.)

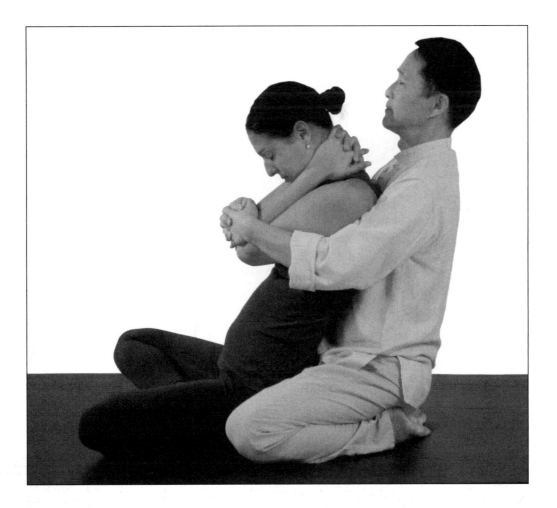

Tea Kettle Twists

- In the Open Archer stance, fix your right knee on the recipient's left leg to stabilize her thigh.
- Place the recipient's left hand on her ear.
- Use your right hand to hold her left elbow.
- Use your left hand to catch the recipient's right triceps with her arm resting on your left leg.
- Push the recipient's left elbow while pulling on the right arm, creating a delicious sideways stretch to the neck and side of the body.

Variations: Continue by rising up into an Open Warrior and with forward rock, give a forward bend spinal twist. Bring the client back up. Now create a sitting spinal twist and open the pectorals through pushing the left elbow back and away from you while you pull the right arm toward you.

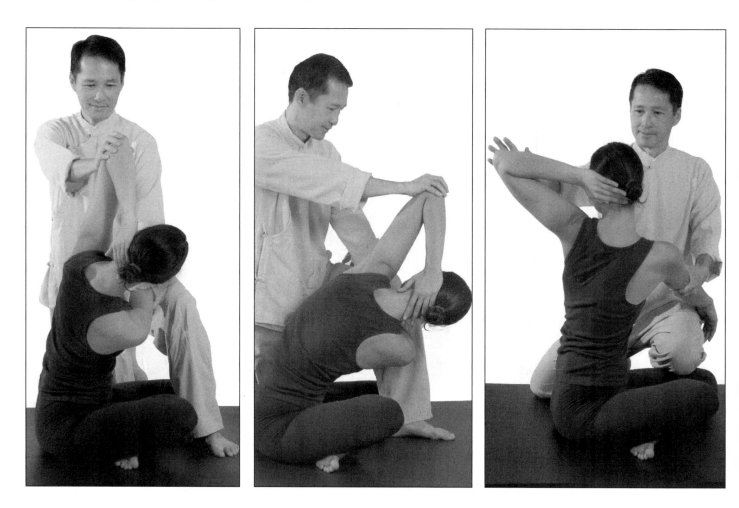

Shoulder Heaven

- Sit in Open Archer facing the client.
- Place your right thumb in the soft spot at the shoulder socket.
- Apply pressure while applying gentle traction by pulling on the arm with your left hand, elbow bent.
- Hold for a count of five.
- Release and repeat twice more.
- Finally, give the arm a swirl, shaking it out in a circular motion (similar to turning the end of a jump rope) while maintaining the pressure with the thumb.

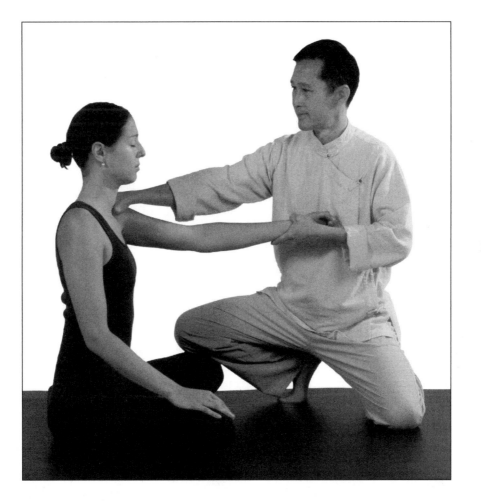

Shoulder Squeeze

- ◆ Sit in Open Archer with your left leg fixed on the recipient's left thigh.
- ◆ Join your palms at the front and back of the recipient's shoulder.
- ◆ Bring your elbows down, lean in slightly, and squeeze.
- ◆ While you squeeze, give the shoulders an upward lift.
- ◆ Continue by lifting the upper arm with your left arm interlaced under her arm, keep your front leg in Archer in place, moving back behind her.
- ◆ Place your left thumb on the recipient's soft spot between the scapula and the spine. Apply pressure and circulate, "greasing" the recipient's shoulder joint.

Note: Before moving on to the next posture, repeat the Tea Kettle Twists, Shoulder Heaven, and Shoulder Squeeze on the other side of the body.

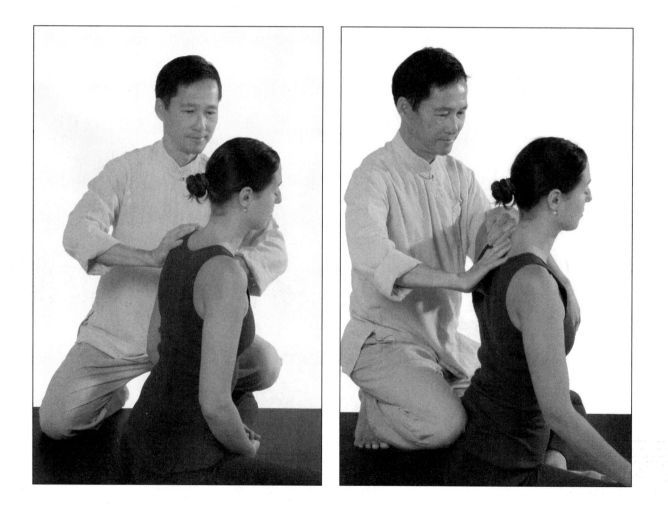

Super Stretch

- ♦ In Kneeling Diamond stance, bring the recipient's arms to her sides and support her shoulders.
- ♦ Sit behind the recipient with your knees bent, continuing to support her with one of your arms.
- ♦ Place the balls of your feet on either side of the sacrum.
- ♦ Support her as she leans back, allowing her to rest on your shins.
- ♦ Hold on to her biceps while extending your legs, allowing her to roll up and rest on the balls of your feet.
- ♦ Bring her hands so that they hold your waist while you hold her arms.
- ♦ Ask the recipient to extend her legs.
- ♦ Lean back for a long extension.
- ♦ To release, bring her arms to the side. Hold her head and lift your knees, cross your legs, and glide out.

Variation: While holding the stretch, make circles with the balls of your feet.

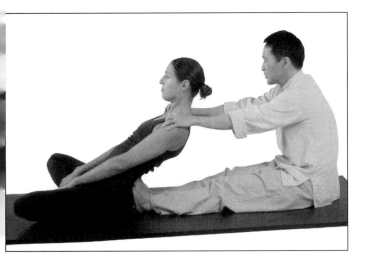
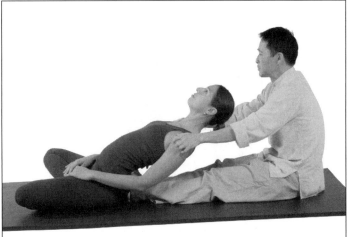
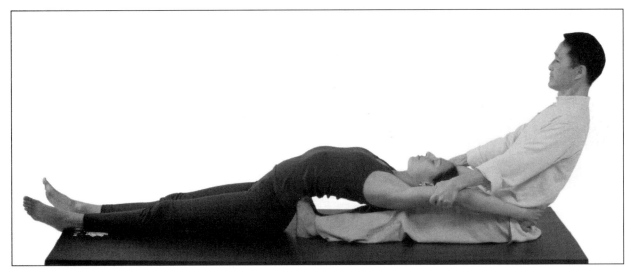

Chin Lock

- Sit behind your recipient. Raise the recipient's head with your palms.
- Gently guide her chin toward the base of her throat.
- Cross your forearms and place your palms, still under the recipient's head, on her shoulders.
- To execute this dynamic move, gently lift the head toward the chest by lifting up both arms.
- Release by gently holding on to the recipient's head and lowering it back down.

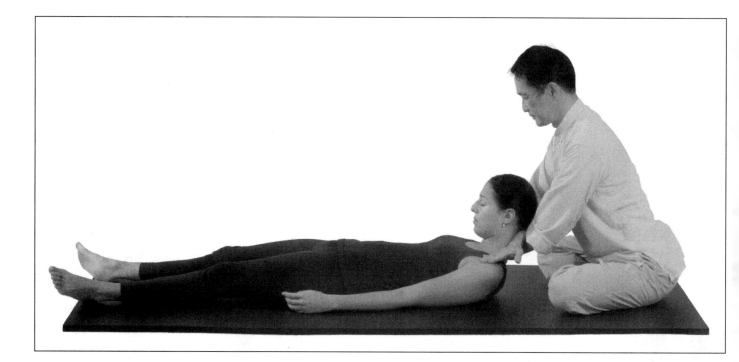

❀ SINGLE LEG POSTURES

These postures can be quite enjoyable, but they are also quite challenging and demand well-developed body-centering skills. Begin these postures on one side of the body and perform the entire sequence before switching to the other side.

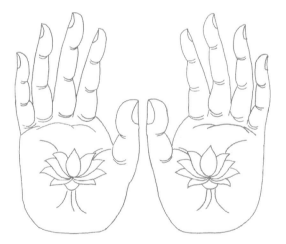

*Indicates postures taught in Lotus Palm's most advanced course, Thai Yoga Massage 6.

Single Foot Blood Stop

- ♦ Stand between the recipient's thighs.
- ♦ Raise your right foot and place your instep one palm-length below the groin across her inner thigh.
- ♦ You may lean your hand on your right leg to help apply pressure.
- ♦ With much control, apply gradual pressure with your foot and sustain for 30–60 seconds.

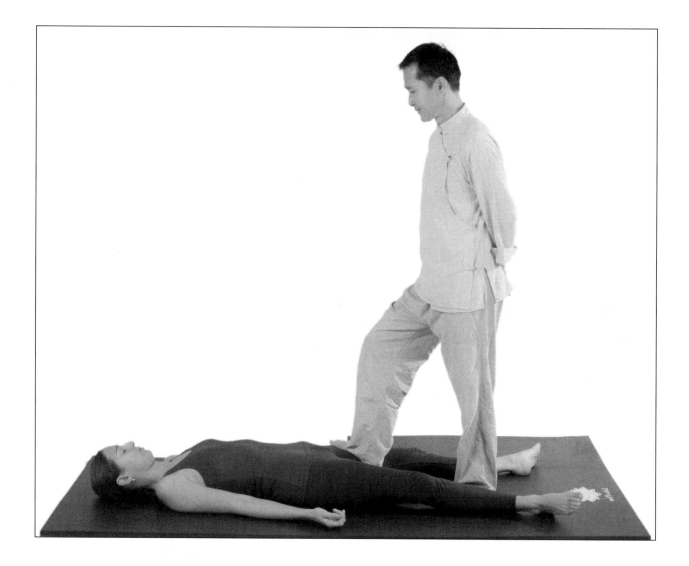

Walking on Sen

- ◆ Stand between the recipient's legs.
- ◆ Place the ball of your foot on the fleshy part of the inner leg, with your heel resting on the mat.
- ◆ Use forward rock to apply pressure.
- ◆ Continue moving up and down the leg.
- ◆ For the upper thigh, stand with your passive leg on the outside of the recipient's legs to complete the posture.

Precaution: With all standing techniques, it's important to have good control and balance. Make sure to check your posture throughout.

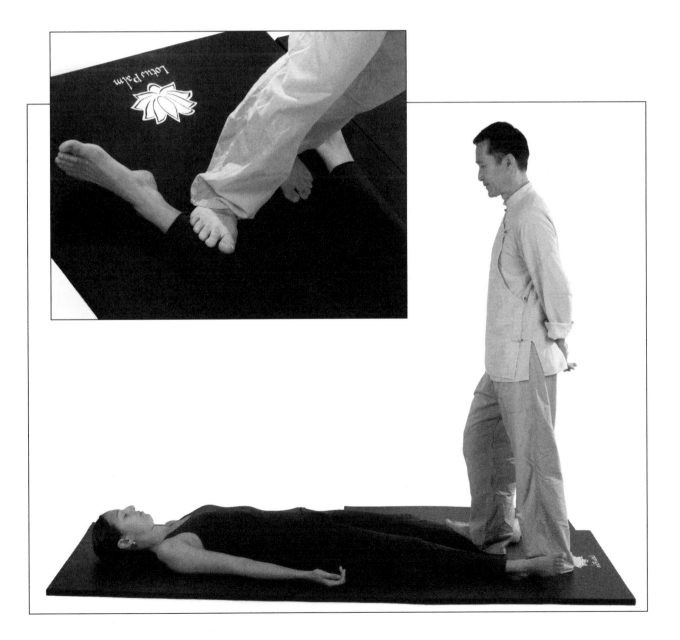

Kneeing on Inner Leg

+ Sit in the Diamond on Toes stance.
+ Place your right hand on the recipient's left leg and left hand on her right shin.
+ Place your knee on the inside leg, remaining on the fleshy part of the leg.
+ Use gradual pressure as you knee up and down the leg.
+ Bring the leg farther out to the side to continue working on the upper leg.

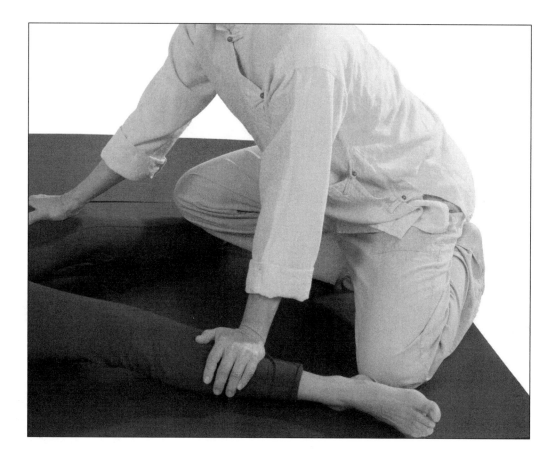

Quad Rock 'n' Roll

- ♦ In a slight Open Diamond, place the recipient's foot between your knees.
- ♦ Interlace your fingers together above her knee on her thigh.
- ♦ With arms straight, lean back, then release, and repeat a few times moving fingers farther down the thigh toward her hip.

Precaution: Avoid placing heels too close to the gluteus maximus (large muscle in the buttocks). This can cause the ankle to hyperextend.

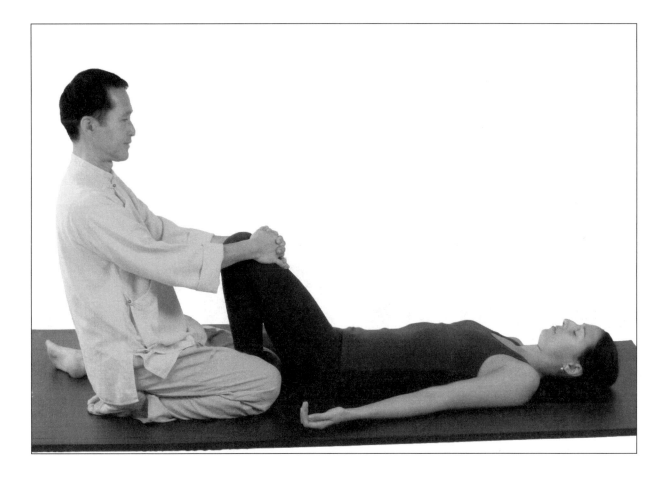

Half Mini AG

♦ Staying in Diamond, place the recipient's foot on your knee.

♦ With your fingers interlaced above her knee on her thigh, lean back with straight arms.

♦ Release and repeat twice more.

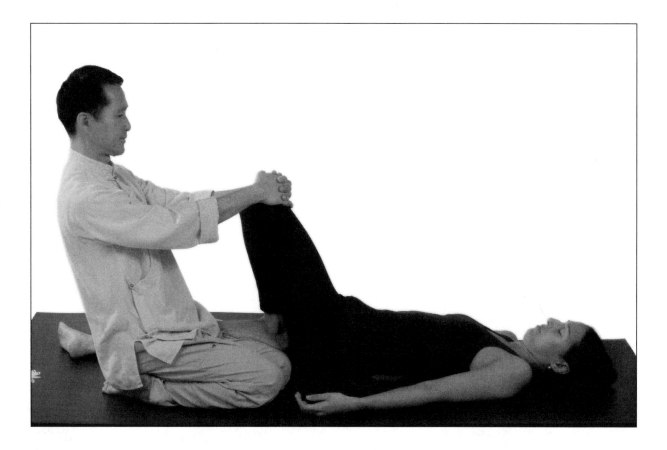

Hamstring Press

- ♦ Come into Archer and place your knee behind the recipient's hamstring.
- ♦ Place recipient's leg on your thigh with the foot hanging next to your hip.
- ♦ Interlace your fingers around her knee.
- ♦ With arms straight, lean back.
- ♦ Release and repeat, positioning your knee down and up the hamstring each time.

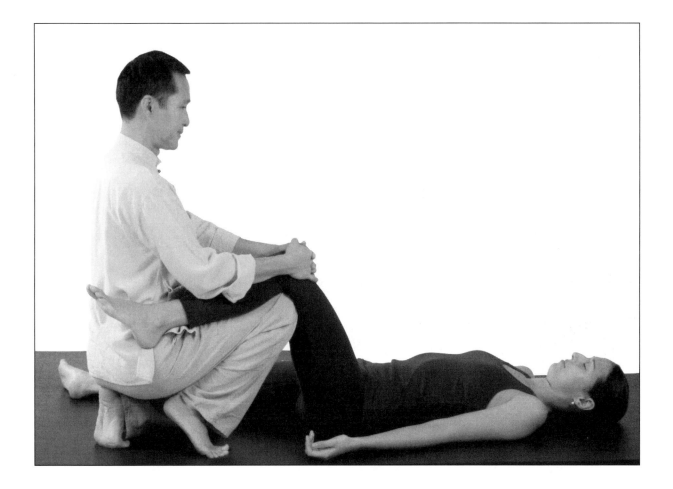

Pigeon Stretch

- ♦ Hold the recipient's leg and move into Warrior.
- ♦ Place your wrist on your Warrior knee, holding the recipient's knee in that hand.
- ♦ With your other hand, hold the recipient's ankle or sole.
- ♦ With your arm straight, pull the knee by gradually twisting your body and shoulders.

Precaution: Avoid pulling too much as this can be a powerful stretch for some.

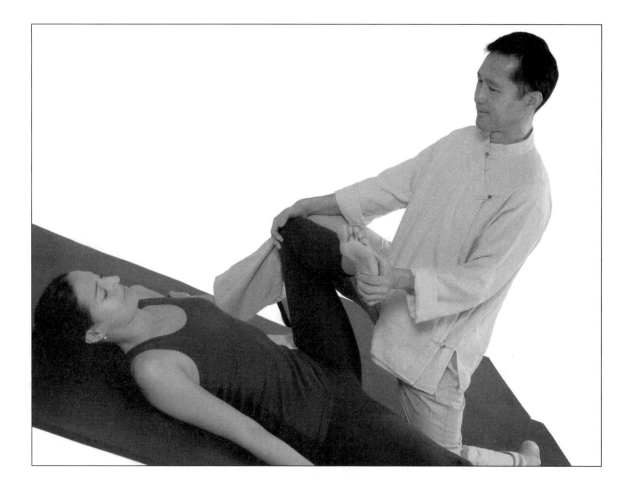

Vishnu Twist

- ♦ Place recipient's foot on the mat above the knee of the leg that is on the ground.
- ♦ Place yourself on the other side of the recipient's body, facing her raised knee.
- ♦ In a slight Open Diamond, place the recipient's foot between your knees.
- ♦ Interlace your fingers behind her knee.
- ♦ Lean back, release, and repeat a few times.

Precaution: Make sure that your knee is anchored above the recipient's knee that is on the mat. Avoid bone on bone contact and place a small cushion between your knee and the side of the recipient's leg.

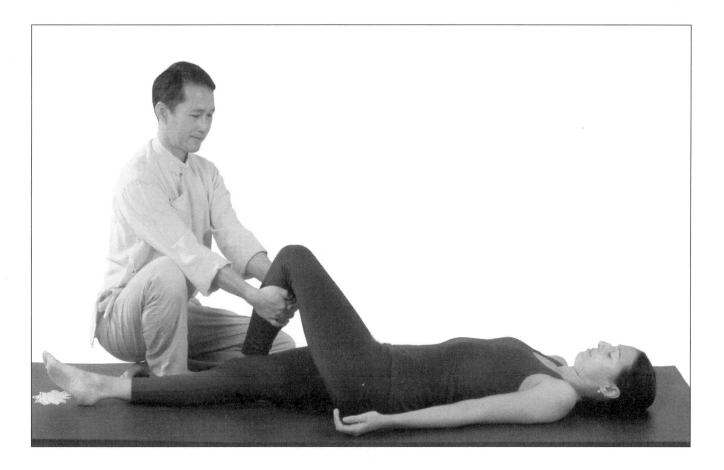

Protractor Kick

- Straighten the recipient's leg across her body at as close to a 90° angle as is comfortable.
- Hold her ankle and position yourself so that you are sitting level with her body.
- Place your right foot in the crease of her far iliac crest and pull.

Precaution: Make sure the heel of your foot is in the crease and not lower on the bladder or stomach.

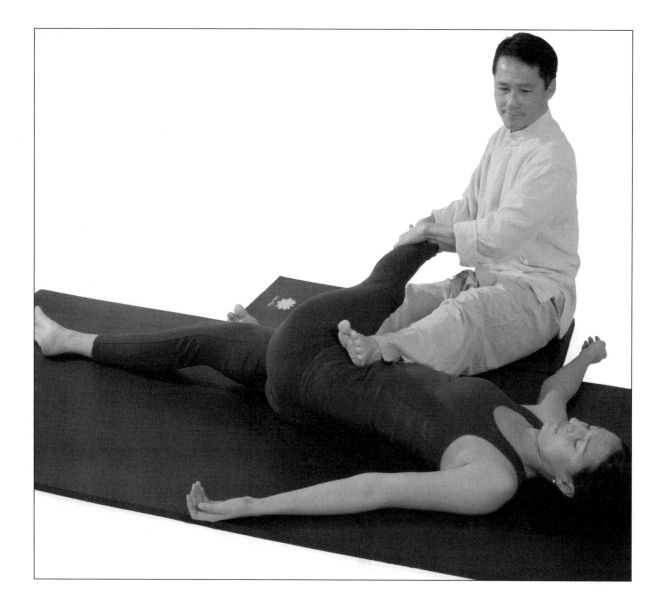

Single Leg Pull

- ♦ Come down to recipient's feet in a Diamond stance.
- ♦ Anchor the recipient's foot (the one you are not working on) against your knee.
- ♦ With both hands, take hold of the ankle and leg on the other side, and lean back.
- ♦ Repeat three times.

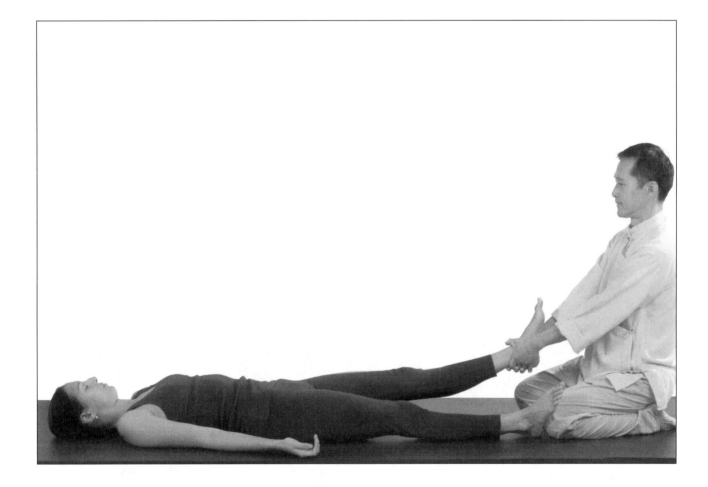

Hurricane Variations

Posture variations help cater to different presenting issues—be it limited mobility, hyperflexibility, body size, or any other question of comfort—so that we can achieve a similar effect with different bodies.

Double Foot Hurricane

- ♦ Sit on the mat between the recipient's legs and bring her leg into an "L" position, flat against the floor and bent at the knee. (If the knee doesn't reach the floor, you can place a pillow under it.)
- ♦ Place your right instep behind her knee and left instep on the thigh.
- ♦ Hold the extended leg with your left hand and the ankle of the bent leg with your right hand (or vice versa).
- ♦ Walk both of your feet up and down her thigh. Pull on the bent leg with your hand to maintain the position.

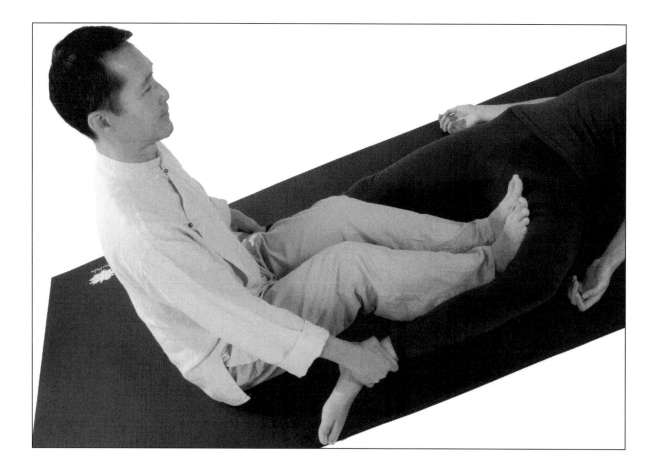

Hurricane Squeeze

- From the Double Foot Hurricane, scoop forward and lock the recipient's foot around both your feet so that her dorsal is wrapped around your left shin.
- Hold the knee with your right hand, and use your left hand to roll the quadriceps muscles toward you.
- Cup your palm and tap the quads to release tension.

Precautions: Make sure your foot that is close to the knee is not right behind the knee. Make sure the gastrocnemius (calf muscle) is exposed, so as not to be squeezed too much.

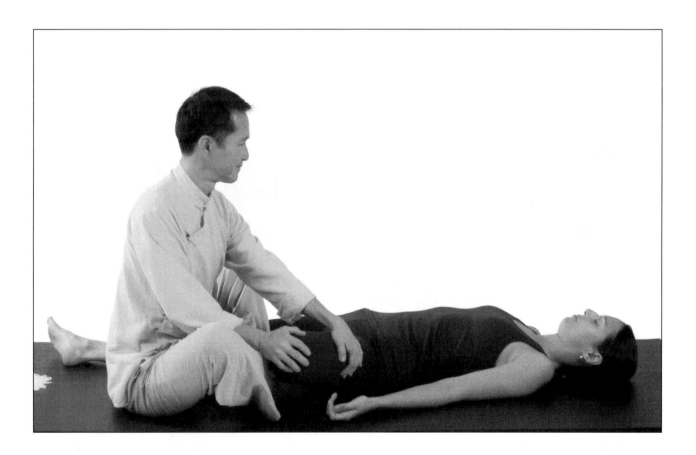

Hurricane Dance

♦ Place your left foot on the recipient's inner thigh and your right foot on the other side of the leg on her quadriceps.

♦ Push with your left and pull with your right.

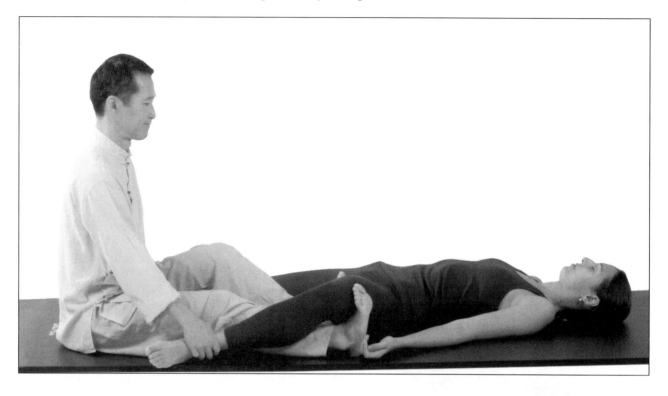

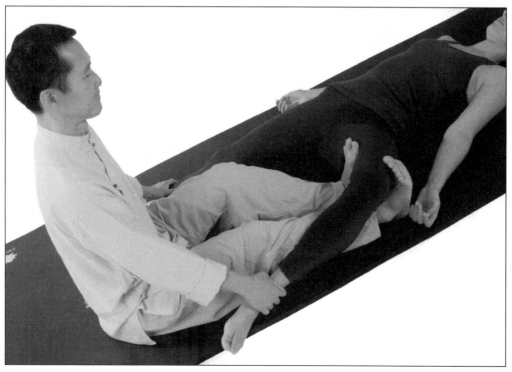

Side Kick Dance

- From the Hurricane Dance, gently kick her Achilles tendon out so the leg is fully extended, and move to the outside of the leg.
- Place her Achilles on the top of your foot and your right instep on her quadriceps.
- Pull back with your left foot while you walk up and down the quad with your right.
- Continue by placing your instep directly on the hip as you pull and push.
- If the recipient is flexible enough, use your hand to pull on the leg and add delicious circles.

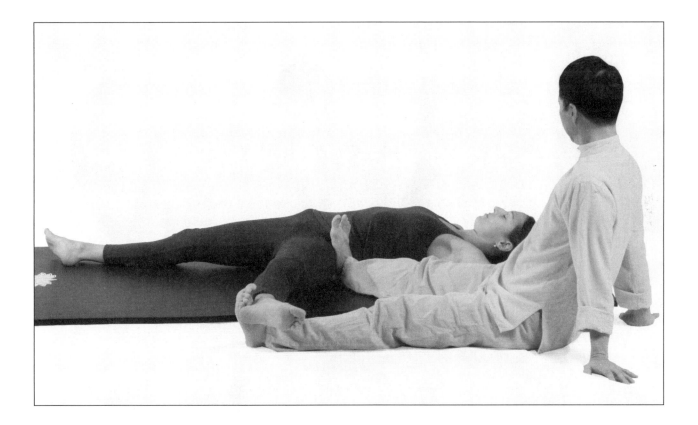

Single Leg Extensions

- ♦ Sit in Diamond pose next to the recipient's leg.
- ♦ Lift your knee up in Warrior and bend her knee, pressing the knee toward her chest, then raise her foot to the ceiling.
- ♦ Keep pushing the raised heel with your right hand while pressing gently on the straight leg on the mat with your left.

Variations: Use your right hand to palm on the back of the thigh while the other pushes on the heel.

For a deeper stretch you can push the heel of the extended leg and also apply pressure with your knee on the hamstring.

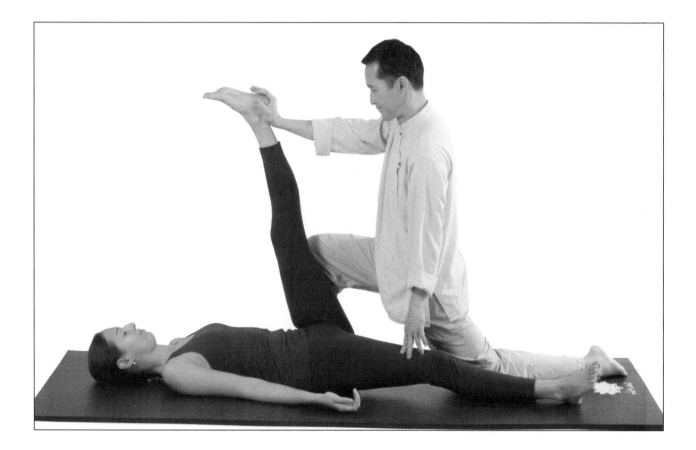

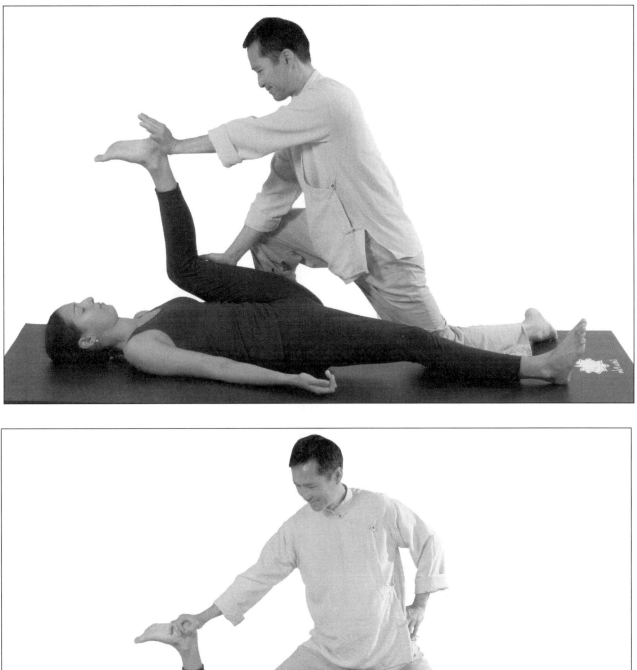

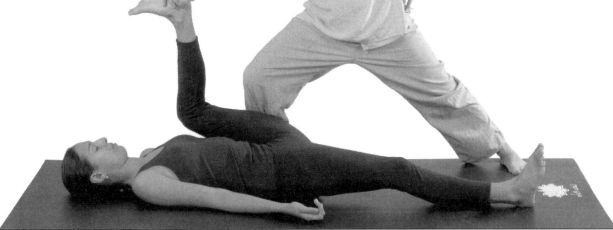

Wish Bone

- From Warrior stance, push the knee toward the recipient's abdomen, then push it over slightly toward the opposite side (creating a light spinal torsion).
- Placing your right foot beneath her left buttocks, turn your foot so that the recipient's sacrum fits into the arch of your foot.
- Gently bring her leg back toward center and fit her knee under your thigh as you pass over it in order to sit your right buttocks upon her inner thigh, which is now resting upon your calf.
- This posture is quite strong, but you may palm on the recipient's opposite hip and thigh with your left hand if you wish to intensify it.

Variation: Instead of your foot, place a pillow under the buttock and press the knee down toward the mat.

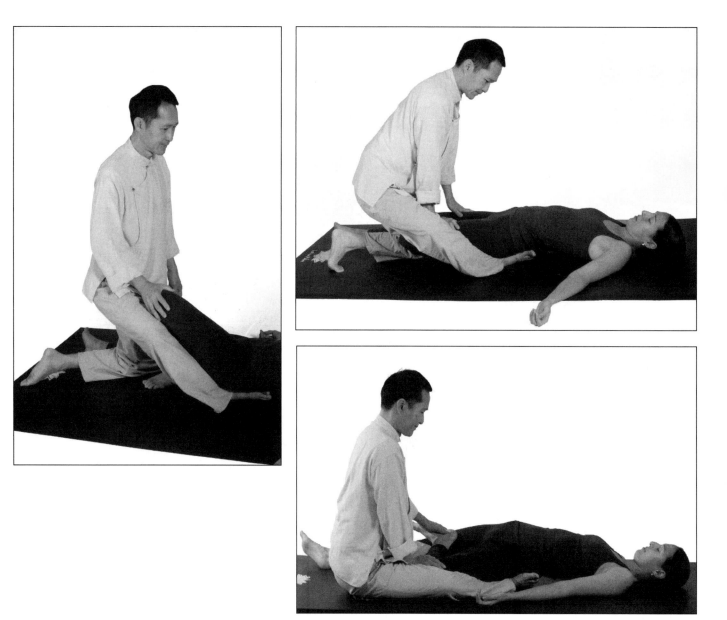

Hip Swing

♦ Step into Warrior stance perpendicular to your client.

♦ Allow her lower leg to rest over your bent, upraised leg.

♦ Raise her hip by leaning your body slightly toward the direction of her foot. This gives traction to the hip and raises the lower back.

♦ Continue by gently swinging her leg.

Repeat this Single Leg Postures series on the other side.

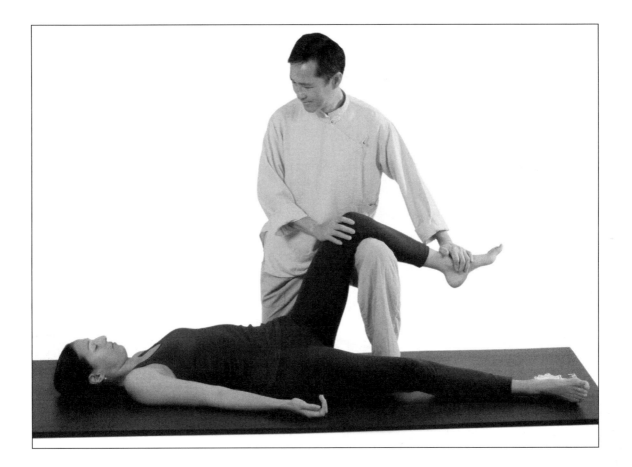

❁ SIDE POSITION POSTURES

Begin this posture series on one side of the body and perform the entire sequence before switching to the other side.

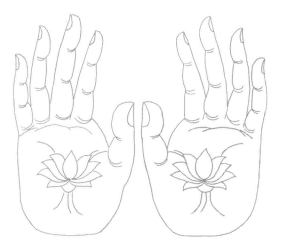

*Indicates postures taught in Lotus Palm's most advanced course, Thai Yoga Massage 6.

Side Sole Walk

- ◆ Starting at the toes, use forward rock to walk all along the recipient's extended foot. The only part of her foot you should avoid is the heel.
- ◆ For added pressure you can turn around and use your heel.

Precaution: In order to help maintain your balance, it is important to prepare a level surface.

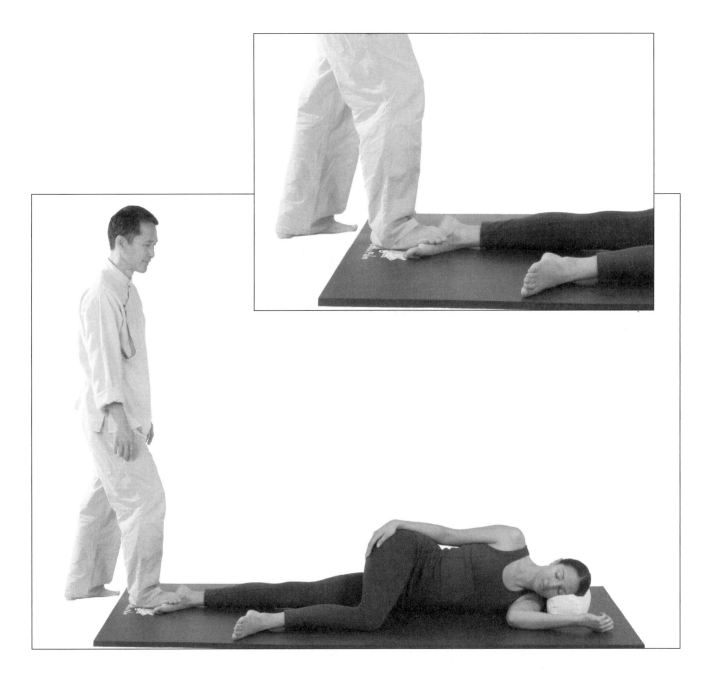

Side Hurricane Dance

- ◆ Sit between the recipient's legs and place both of your feet at the back of her thigh.
- ◆ Wrap her foot so it's locked on the outside of your left shin.
- ◆ Use your two hands to squeeze the quadriceps. Continue by tapping.

Precaution: Make sure to release the gastrocnemius (calf) muscle to avoid any pinching or discomfort.

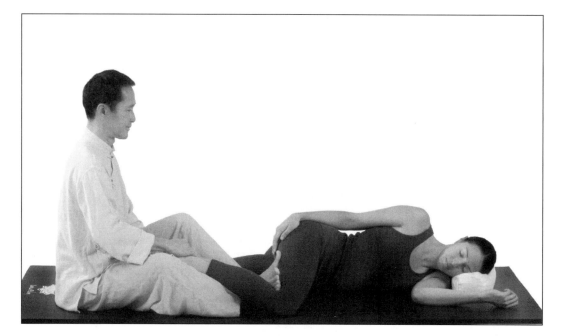

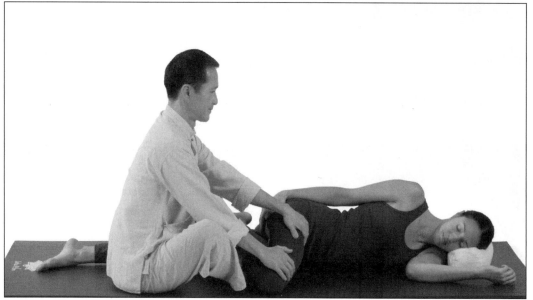

Kneeling Leg Fold

- ♦ Place yourself in Warrior over your recipient's straight leg.
- ♦ With both hands on her foot, bring up her leg, bending it and placing her upper leg on the thigh of your raised leg.
- ♦ Your right hand is on her knee while you push her leg toward her buttocks.

Variations: For a stronger stretch, fix the leg in between your thigh and her buttock, and use two hands on the knee to pull back.

For the strongest version, step out into Open Archer to lean back even farther.

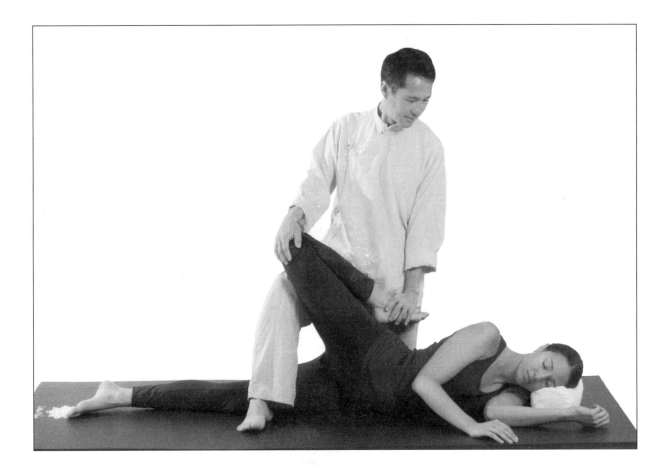

Back Walk

- ◆ Sit behind the recipient, perpendicular to her back.
- ◆ Place your left hand on her wrist, gently pulling and twisting her toward you, and hold the ankle of the extended leg closest to you with your right hand.
- ◆ Place your feet above the sacrum and pull on the leg while you walk on the back and the thigh.

Variation: You can hold either of the recipient's legs or both, depending on your preference.

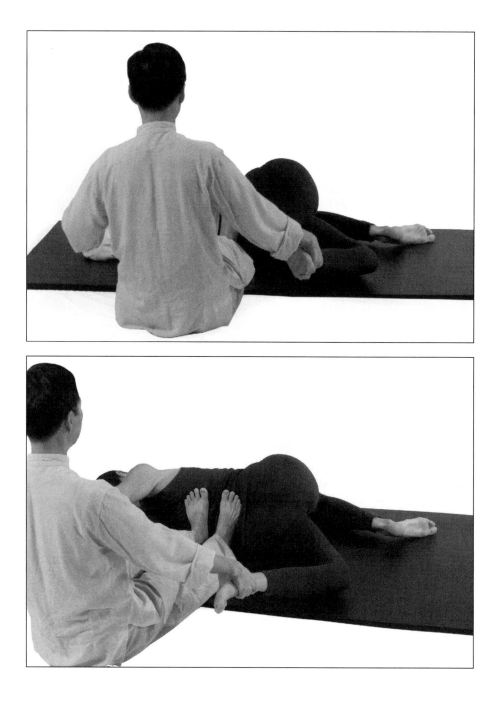

Dead Man Twist

+ Cross the recipient's right arm over her left.
+ Stand with your feet a little wider than shoulder-width apart in Horse Riding stance, with your feet straddling the recipient's straight leg, just behind her buttocks.
+ Bend your knees and take the recipient's left wrist with both your hands.
+ Straighten your legs and lift the recipient off the ground, instructing her to relax if necessary.

Variation: Knee into the buttock while holding on to the wrist. (No need to lift the person off the ground.)

Precaution: This exercise should be done without any jerky movements. This posture is not suited for recipients who have had any prior arm or shoulder injuries. Go easy! As the practitioner, avoid performing this posture on clients who are much heavier than you in order to protect your back.

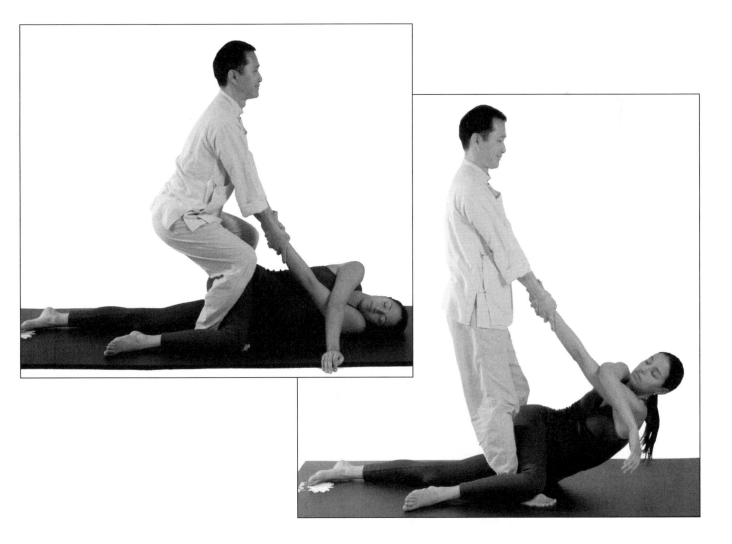

Side Tea Pot and Chicken Wing Roll

- ♦ Move into Kneeling Diamond alongside the recipient's body.
- ♦ Bend the recipient's arm and place her palm on her ear.
- ♦ Place your left hand on her elbow and your right hand on her hip.
- ♦ Create a nice side extension. Hold for a count of five, release and repeat.
- ♦ For the Chicken Wing Roll, extend the recipient's arm above her head and roll your forearm along the side of her body and around the "chicken wing" area of the back (so aptly named by Kam Thye!).

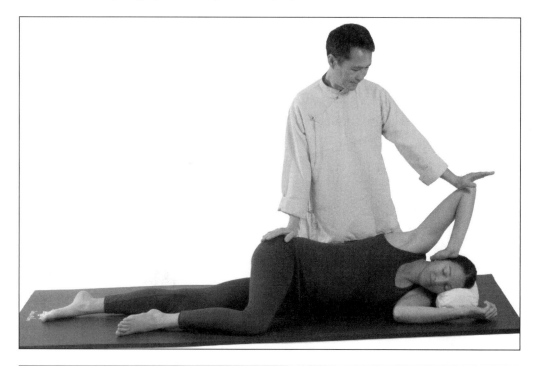

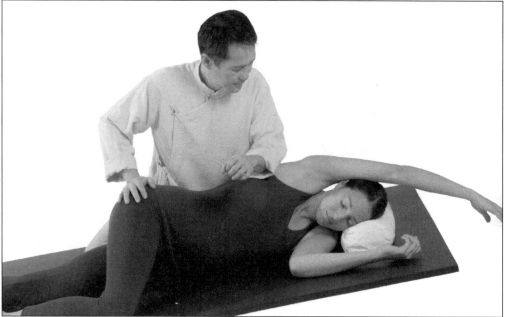

Side Arm Extension

- ♦ Still in Kneeling Diamond behind the recipient, lift her arm and squeeze all along it.
- ♦ Finally, give the arm good traction, lifting with two hands on the wrist.

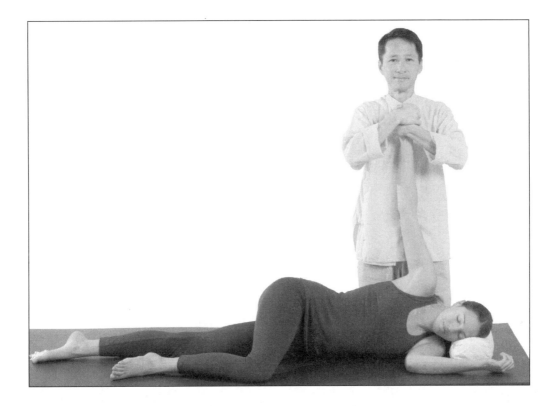

Shoulder Swing

- ◆ Place yourself in Warrior over the recipient's body and place her arm over your thigh to create traction.
- ◆ Lean gradually to your right to increase the stretch.
- ◆ Use your left hand to squeeze the bicep and triceps.

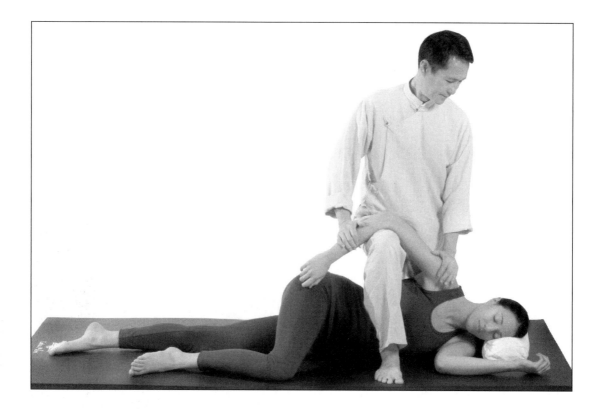

Divine Neck Massage

There are many techniques you can add to a neck massage sequence on the side. Two of our favorites are Jade Pillow and Scap-pulla.

- ♦ To begin, seat yourself in Diamond parallel to your recipient.
- ♦ Interlace your left arm under hers in a nice embrace and practice shoulder rotations (not shown).
- ♦ For the side Jade Pillow, begin by massaging along the ridge where the head meets the neck (at the occipital bone). Move from behind the ear toward the center of the head.
- ♦ For the side Scap-pulla, use the circular motion of shoulder rotations to place your left fingers under the scapula. Gently massage as you make circles with her shoulder.

Repeat this Side Position Postures series on the other side.

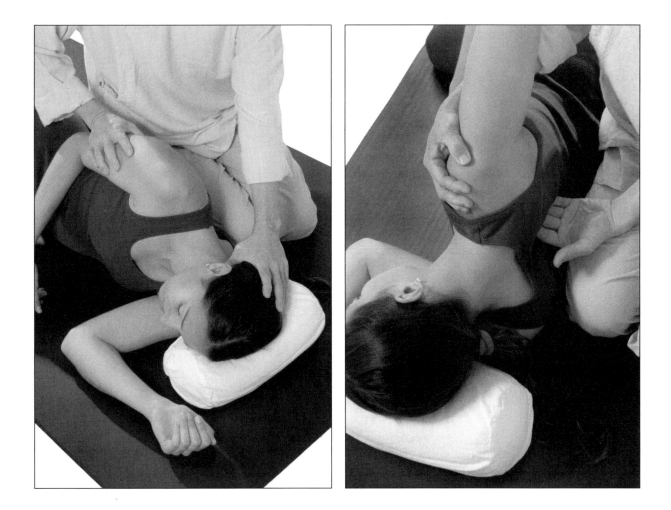

❁ BACK POSTURES

The back is the most requested area for massage, and work on this area is highly beneficial for the body. Place a small pillow under the recipient's forehead to keep the nose from being pushed into the mat. If the recipient prefers to turn the head to one side, periodically request that it be turned to the other side, to avoid stiffness in the neck.

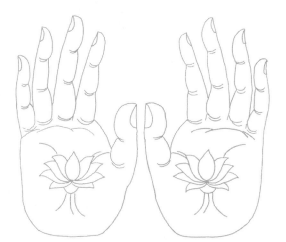

---

*Indicates postures taught in Lotus Palm's most advanced course, Thai Yoga Massage 6.

Hamstring Walk

- ♦ Open the recipient's knees a little wider than side by side.
- ♦ Place your instep behind her knee.
- ♦ Use gradual pressure as you step onto the back of the leg.

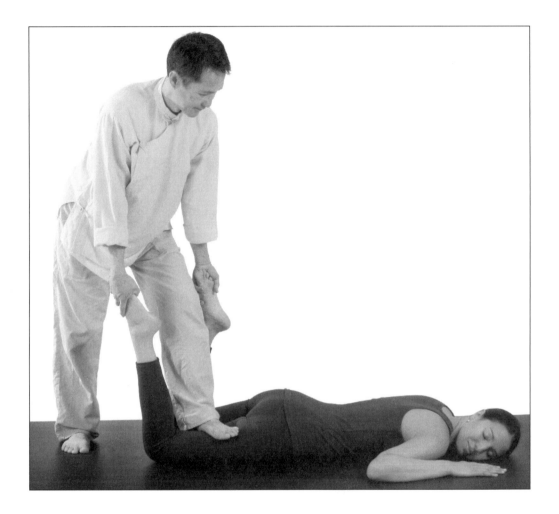

Palming the Back in Hamstring

- ♦ Step onto both hamstrings, on the back of the leg above the knees.
- ♦ Lock the recipient's feet around your legs.
- ♦ Lean forward and palm the back.
- ♦ To release, simply raise up and step off.

Precaution: To keep your balance, place one hand on the sacrum before you step on the second hamstring. Use the same technique when coming off.

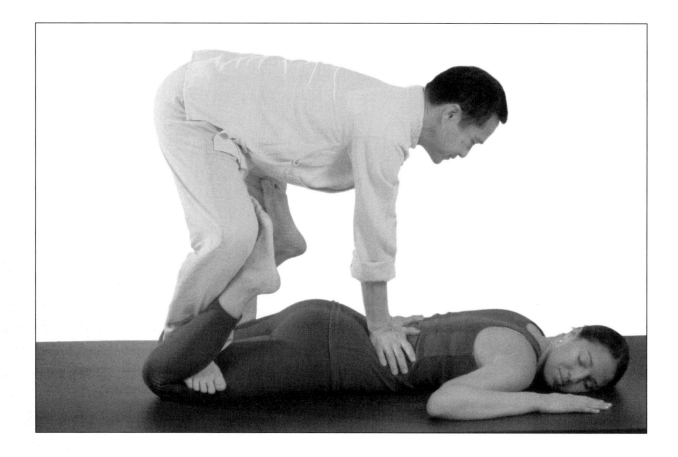

Chakra Asanas

- ♦ Bend the recipient's knees so that her feet come up and create a flat seat for you.
- ♦ Sit on the balls of her feet and find your balance.
- ♦ Bring her arms up and rest her palms on your upper legs.
- ♦ Start by palming her back with forward rock, with your back and arms straight.

Variation: Continue with shoulder opening and scapula pull. Wrap your outside hand around the shoulder and place your thumb in between the scapula and spine, working your way up the back.

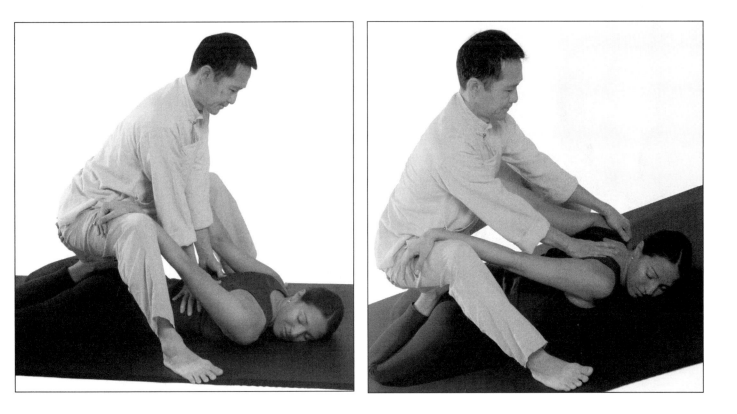

Complete Chakra Pose

- Bring your hands to the recipient's armpits, grasping her shoulders.
- Direct your recipient to inhale, and as she exhales, bring her up, supporting her arms on your thighs.

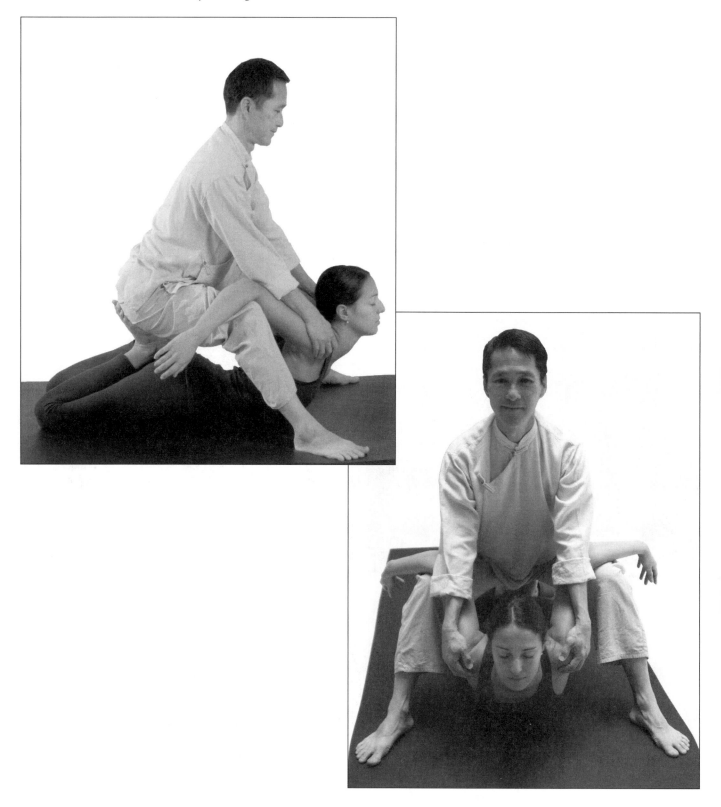

Sanuk Variations

Sanuk "Orange Press"

- In Sanuk,* place your right forearm behind the knee and bend the recipient's leg so her foot goes toward her buttocks.
- Rock in and squeeze.

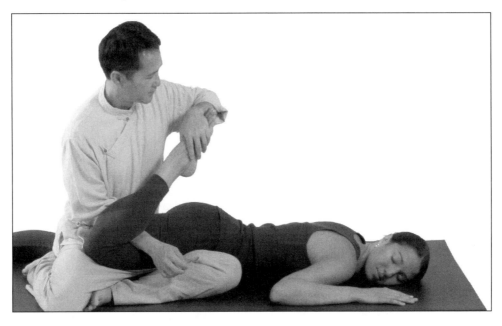

Elbow Traction

- Wrap your arms around the recipient's leg and use your body weight to lean in to the buttocks with your elbow.

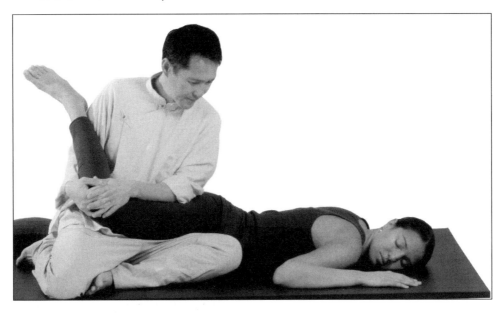

*Complete instructions for Sanuk are provided in *Thai Yoga Massage*, page 109.

Reverse Leg Fold

- ◆ Place yourself in Open Diamond on your toes.
- ◆ Cross the recipient's ankle behind her knee and press the other leg forward using your forward rock.

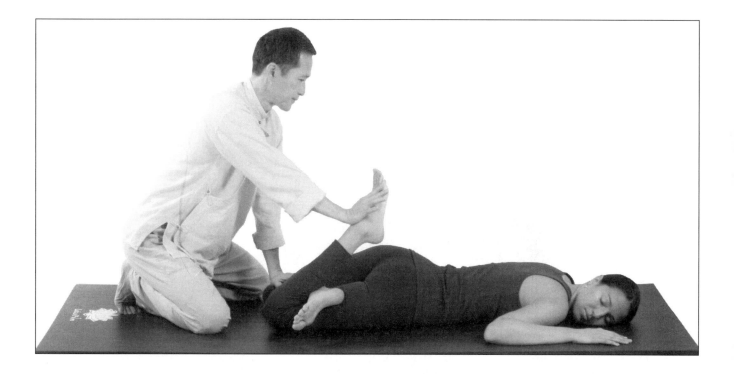

Seated Locust

♦ Place a pillow on the recipient's lower back and sit lightly on her sacrum facing her feet.

♦ Interlace your hands around her extended knee.

♦ Keeping your back straight, gently lean back to apply a backward arc.

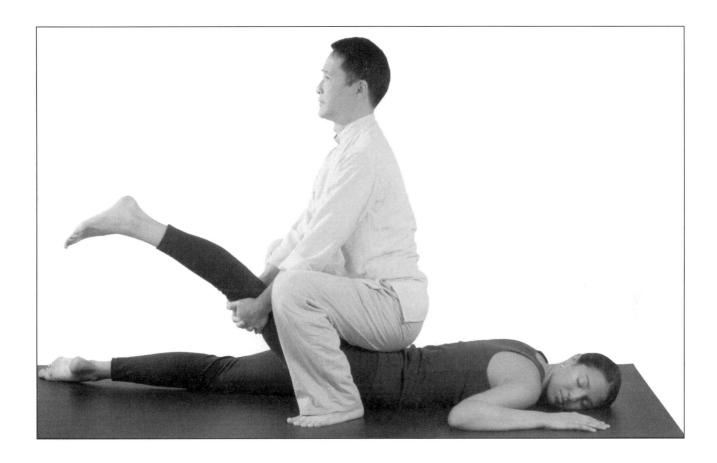

Warrior Scapula

- ◆ Place yourself in Warrior straddled over the recipient's body. Bring her arm onto your upper leg.
- ◆ Use your one hand to hold on to the shoulder.
- ◆ Use the other to thumb in and under the scapula.

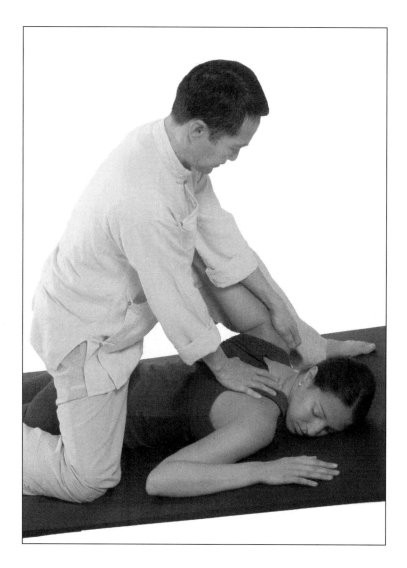

Shoulder Stretch

♦ Seat yourself alongside the body of your recipient in a Half Lotus.

♦ Extend your right leg so that your foot is fixed firmly in her right armpit.

♦ Take her left arm and gently lean back, giving a nice long traction of the shoulder.

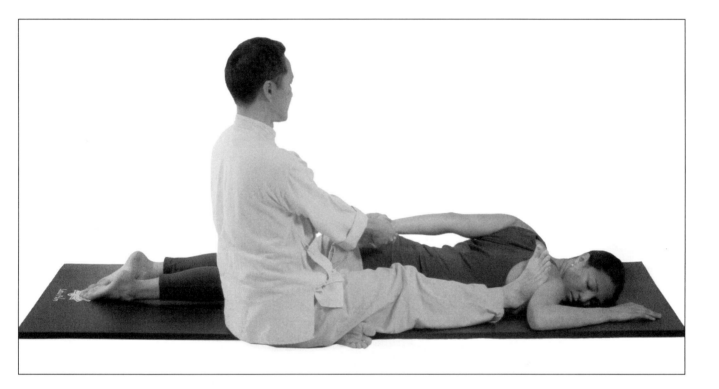

Back Massage Variations
Low Back Points

- Place yourself off to one side of the recipient's low back.
- Use a combination of palming, kneeing, squeezing, and thumbing to massage all along the waistline.
- Change sides and repeat.

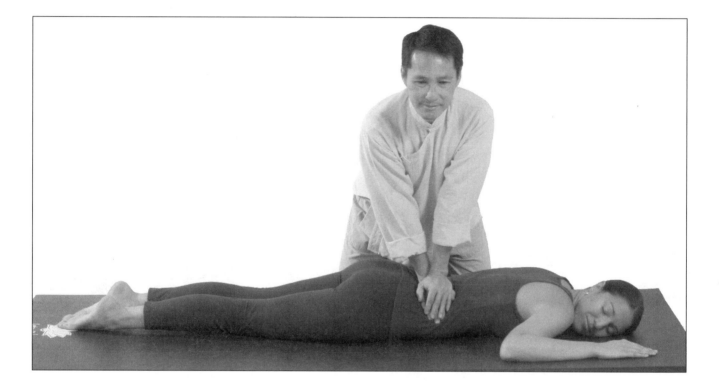

Lobster Claw

+ Put your thumb and fingers on the edge of the recipient's spine.
+ Use firm pressure to rock in while you massage all along the edge of the spine.
+ Repeat on the other side.

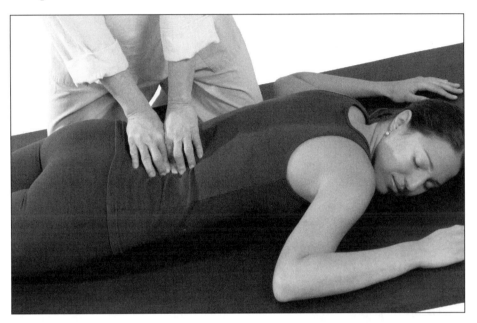

Clamshell

+ Place yourself in Warrior over the recipient's body.
+ Interlace your fingers and gently use your knuckles to rock up and down the body.
+ This is especially effective on the muscles between the scapula and the spine.

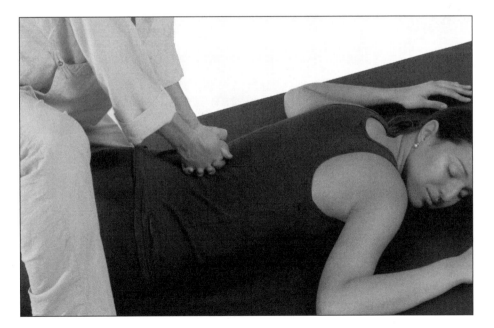

Nutcracker

- Place yourself in Warrior over the recipient's body.
- Place your hands with fingers bent as in a bear claw, knuckles placed firmly on the back.
- Apply pressure and then firmly drop into a fist movement so that you finish by using the knuckles of your fist to apply pressure.

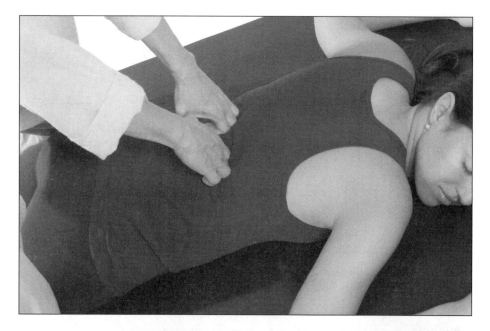

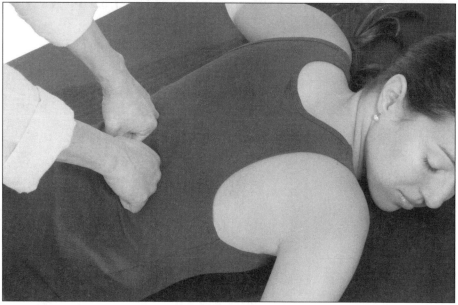

Massage from the Top

♦ A beautiful way to complete your back work is to position yourself at the top of your recipient's body.

♦ From here you can easily reach the shoulders and add in a couple of our other favorites, including:

- Using your elbows to massage the back
- Rising into Downward Dog to palm the lower back and sacrum

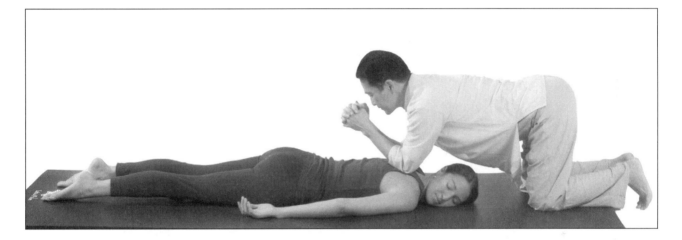

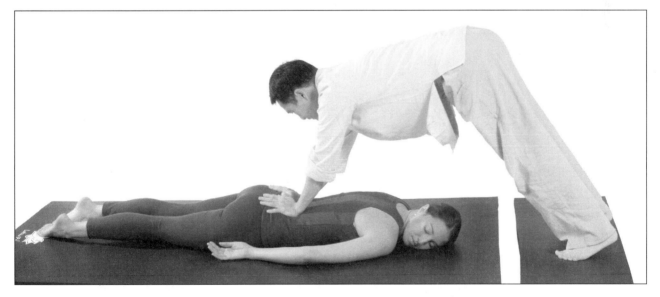

✿ DOUBLE LEG POSTURES

Finding the right distance between you and your recipient will create a seesaw effect when you bring her into a posture, making this posture series almost effortless. Be aware of the alignment of your body, especially your back.

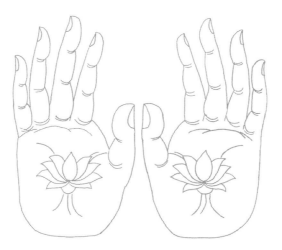

*Indicates postures taught in Lotus Palm's most advanced course, Thai Yoga Massage 6.

Half Shoulder Stand

- Sit in Diamond Stance and hold the recipient's heels.
- Come up to standing with left knee in Warrior, pushing the recipient's heels forward.
- The recipient's legs should be straight.
- Ask her to place her hands on her knees, arms straight and elbows locked.
- Forward rock so that her back comes off the mat.

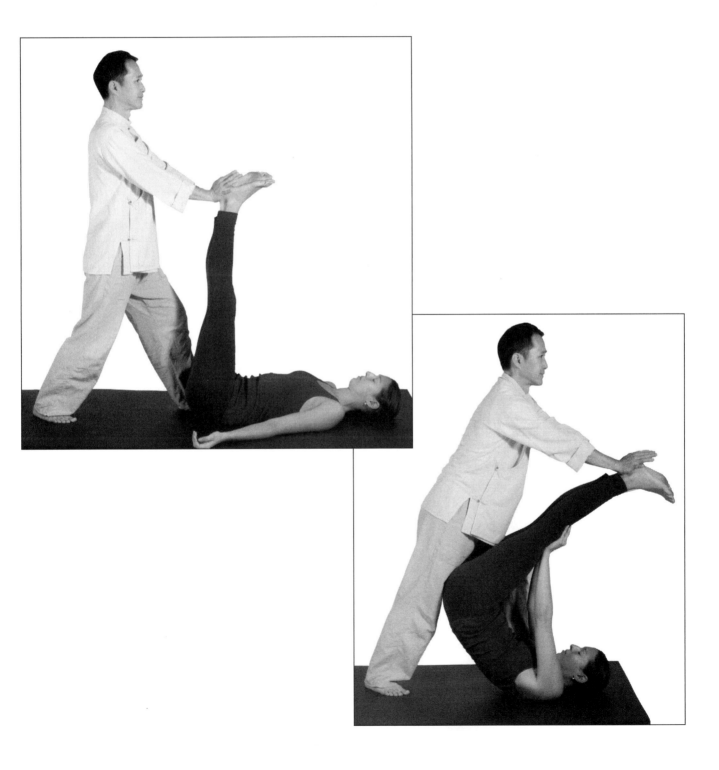

Yoke Variations

♦ Move the recipient into the Yoke posture:
- In Horse Riding stance, bend her left leg.
- Place her left ankle above her right knee.

Forward Bend and Twist

♦ Step forward, moving as high as possible alongside the recipient's body.

♦ Push her straight leg forward.

♦ Add a twist by pushing this extended leg to the opposite side of the body.

♦ Step back to go into Press Release.

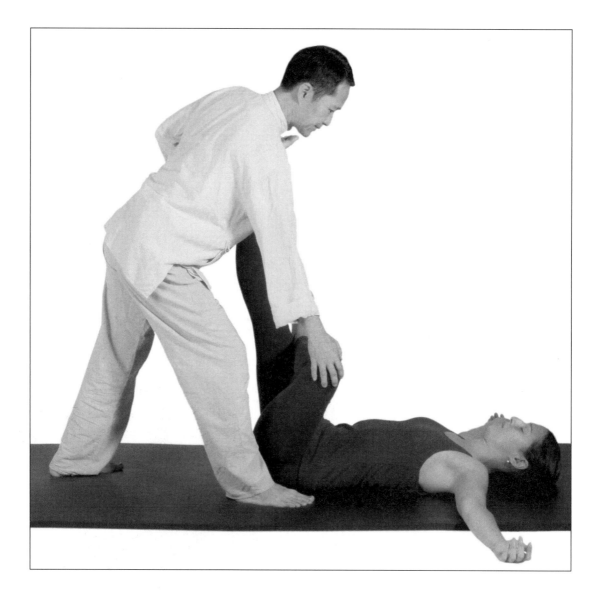

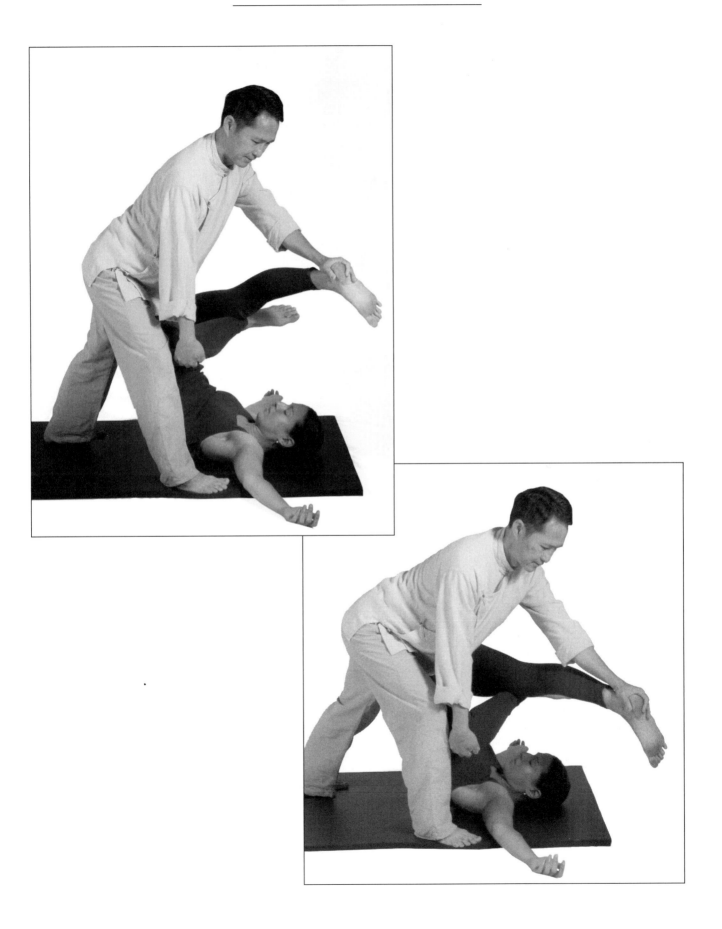

Press Release

- Bring your forward leg in front of the "yoke" of the recipient's bent leg in order to open up the hip.
- Bring the foot of the recipient's straight leg alongside your body and use your forearm or elbow to roll on the sole of her foot. (Using your elbow will allow you to give a deeper massage.)

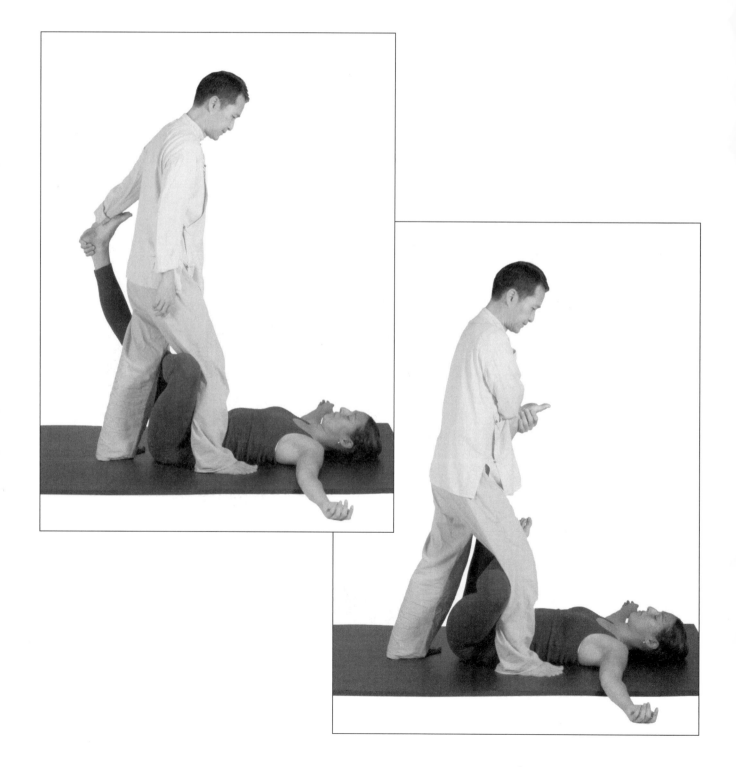

Yoke Twist

- Bring the recipient's straight leg down so it is lying on the mat and her crossed leg down so that the foot is on the mat with the knee pointing up to the ceiling.
- Come into Warrior and use your knee to apply pressure along the back of her bent leg.
- Push the recipient's knee all the way over to the mat on the opposite side.
- Use your left knee to stabilize the hip while you palm the shoulder.

Repeat the Yoke Variations on the other side.

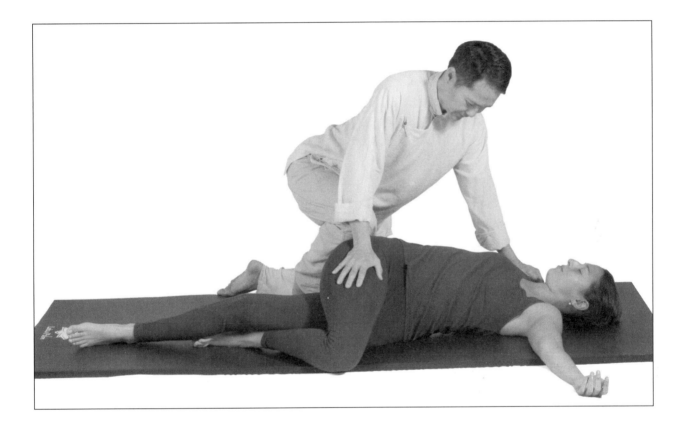

Butterfly Rock

- Open up the legs and step forward in a big Horse Riding stance, straddling the recipient's body.
- Position yourself in front of the recipient's legs with your feet close to her armpits, leaving a small distance between your feet and her body.
- Join her feet together in front of your legs.
- Press her feet downward.
- To add the Butterfly Rock, rock the feet forward.

To release:

- Straighten the legs behind you and take a step back.
- Hold the legs with your left hand, and then do a Sufi Swirl, or circle over the body to come back behind the legs.

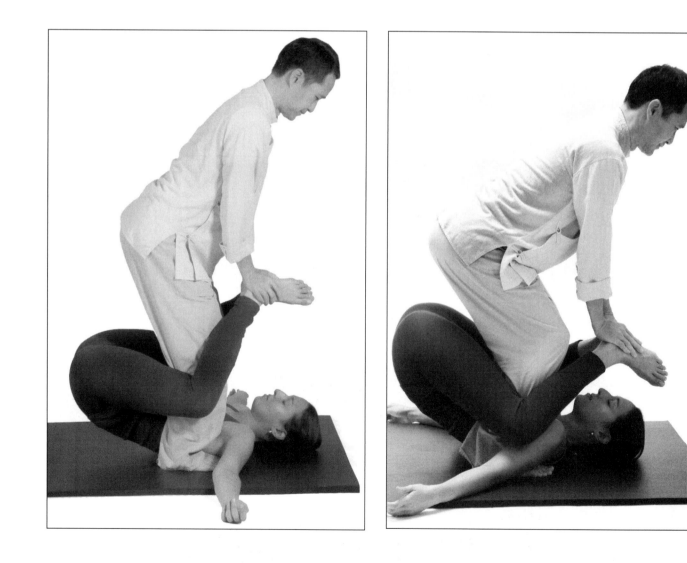

The Sofa

♦ Place a pillow on the recipient's abdomen (not shown).

♦ Place the recipient's feet at the back of your knees and sit on her lower legs.

♦ Begin leaning back by placing your hands on her thighs, and then lay back, all the way down on your recipient.

Precaution: Do not do this on people with hyperextended knees, or those with knee problems.

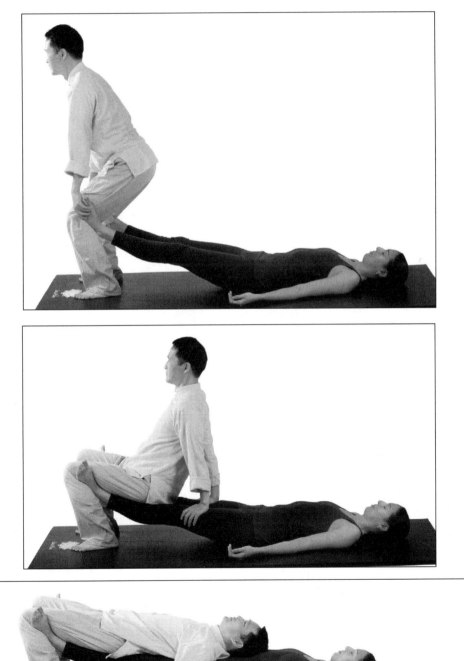

Bridge

- Extend the recipient's legs so they are straight up.
- Hold her ankles and lift her lower body so that you can place your knees on either side of her sacrum.
- Allow her legs to fall to the side as you hold on to her lower back.
- Lower yourself into a squat and she will rise into a backbend.

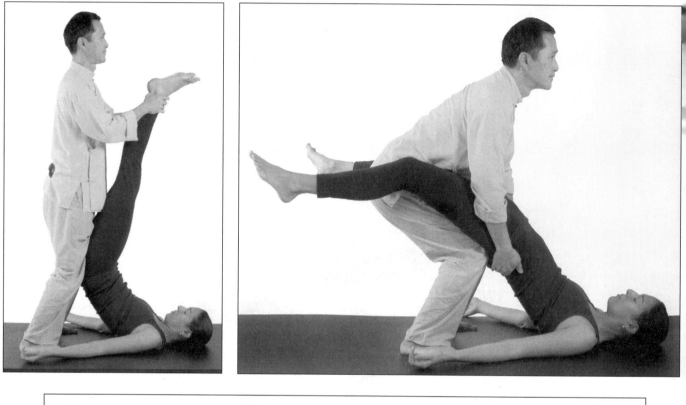

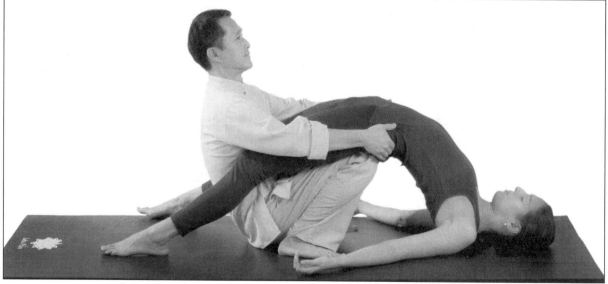

To release:

♦ Ask the recipient to lower her chin toward her chest. You then rise up again to a standing position.

Variation: To reduce the extension, you can instruct your recipient to place her legs on your hips as you bring them down into the Bridge pose.

Precaution: This is a very strong posture which should be performed only on clients in good physical shape, especially as it relates to their back and neck. There are many variations for a lighter backbend.

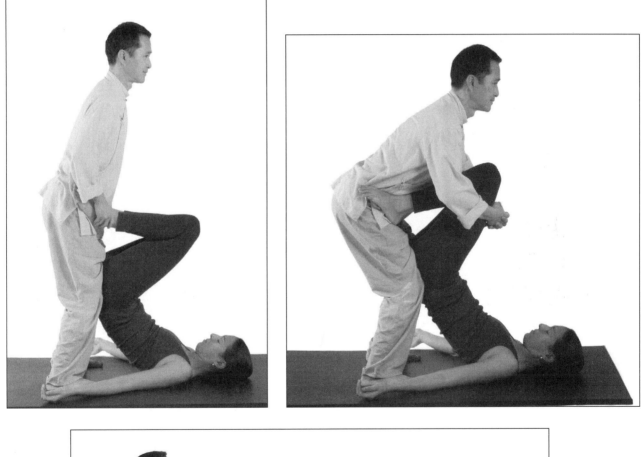

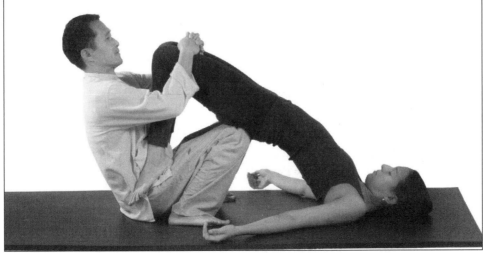

✿ ABDOMEN MASSAGE

The abdomen is a very sensitive part of the body, as well as intimate for some people, so first ask your recipient if she would like to be massaged in this area. Abdomen massage is contraindicated if the recipient is pregnant.

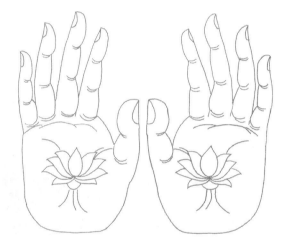

---

*Indicates postures taught in Lotus Palm's most advanced course, Thai Yoga Massage 6.

Ab Massage from the Knees

- ♦ Place your recipient's feet flat on the mat with knees bent and pointed upward.
- ♦ Sit on her knees.
- ♦ Massage the reflex points with your palms.

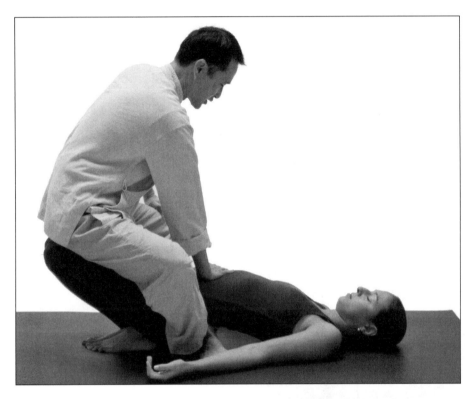

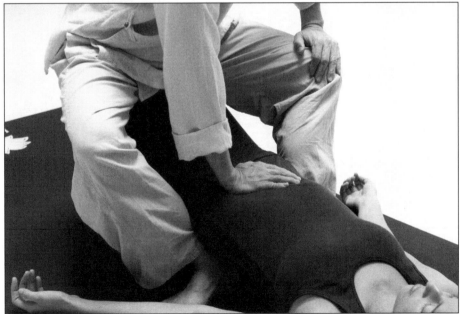

Supported Back Bend

- ♦ Place yourself at the center of your recipient's body.
- ♦ Place your hands on the recipient's hips and gently raise her, taking care to keep your back straight.
- ♦ Bring your legs in to grip the recipient's body and hold her suspended for a count of 5–10 seconds.

Precaution: Take care to perform this posture only with people who are not much heavier than you. Avoid if you have back pain.

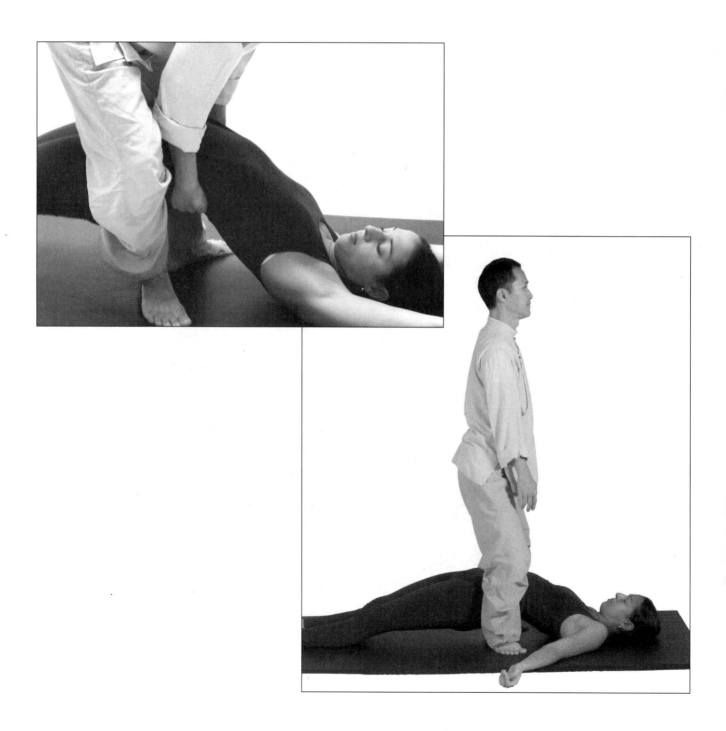

4

Thai Yoga Massage Protocols for Common Ailments

One of the most common scenarios encountered as a therapist is that clients come with a particular problem or pain, and they are looking to massage for an answer. Indeed, there is no doubt that Thai Yoga Massage has many terrific benefits.

Before addressing their issues, a basic understanding of the nature of the discomfort they face is often an integral part of the treatment process. To this end, the three questions you ask at the start of the massage, along with a personal health questionnaire or Ayurvedic consultation that attempts to map a client profile, are integral components of a session—as is a basic understanding of muscle trauma.*

UNDERSTANDING MUSCLE TRAUMA IN THE BODY

The most natural state of the body is movement. Whether subtle or gross, internal or external, we are always engaged in some kind of movement. In fact, about the only time the body is 100 percent relaxed is when we stop breathing. Therefore, when there is muscle pain, the best thing to do is stimulate movement that is appropriate for the individual. Muscles need to be exercised to maintain tone and condition. If allowed to rest for lengthy periods of time, muscles can become weak. Without movement—

---

*Always inquire about physical limitations (Is there any particular movement that you cannot or should not do?) as well as other health issues (other than movement restrictions) and ask if there is a particular part of the body that would like special attention. For more information on Ayurvedic consultations, see *Thai Yoga Therapy for Your Body Type*. For more on muscle trauma, see the following section as well as the appendix.

which is the natural state for muscles—oxygen, nutrients, and waste materials become trapped and can possibly lead to increased pain and more serious trauma or chronic ongoing pain.

When considering muscle trauma and Thai Yoga Massage, there are three important aspects to consider:

- The different ways muscle traumas can present themselves
- Why muscle trauma is so common
- The best Thai Yoga Massage approach to help in treatment of the trauma

Muscles are the body's greatest workhorses, and considering how busy we all are, that's saying a lot! Muscles give us the ability to realize every physical goal the brain can imagine, as well as every function needed to survive and thrive.

Muscles are extremely important because they turn energy into motion. We use our heart muscles for pumping blood, chest muscles for breathing, mouth muscles for speaking, body muscles for movement, and hand muscles for expression. Every idea we generate is put into action through our muscles. And what's so amazing about muscles is that most of them are self-healing and grow stronger the more you use them.

There are three types of muscles in the body:

1. Voluntary muscles of the skeletal system
2. Involuntary smooth muscles (muscles that push food along in the digestive system, focus eyes, control the width of arteries, and so on)
3. Involuntary cardiac muscles (specific to the heart)

Naturally, the main concern as massage therapists is with the first category. There are about 605 skeletal muscles and they make up about half the weight in the body. Muscles work in conjunction with the skeletal and nervous systems. A typical skeletal muscle stretches from one bone to another, crossing at least one joint. Muscles are attached to bones via tendons and/or ligaments. Messages are continually sent through the spinal cord and spinal nerves, which direct your muscles. Each muscle has thousands of fibers that start sliding along each other when stimulated with an electrical impulse, causing a contraction. This contraction causes a muscle to move one bone relative to another.

Invariably over a lifetime people experience some trauma to some of their muscles. The subject of muscle trauma and pain is inexhaustible, but we will identify some key indicators that will help answer your client's questions and influence how you customize the massage.

The most common causes of muscle pain or trauma are:

- Tension or stress
- Overuse: Using a muscle too much, too soon, or too often
- Injury

Some other causes of muscle trauma include:

- Chronic illnesses that develop over time, such as fibromyalgia
- Infections
- Mineral and vitamin imbalance
- Drugs, both pharmaceutical and recreational

Muscle trauma can refer to a wide spectrum of effects to the muscles and their intersection points. Because muscles interact with bones and tendons as well as nerves, there is no clear separation when mentioning the different kinds of trauma that can affect the muscles. Taken in its most general sense, muscle trauma can actually refer to any discomfort, pain, restriction in movement, or chronic condition that muscles experience.

Most often a client will present a problem and look to you for an answer. How often have you heard questions such as, "What is this pain I feel? Why does it happen?" Whether it's a pain in the back, a headache that hasn't gone away for several days, knee pain, or any number of ailments, when there's physical discomfort that needs attention, usually it's a musculoskeletal problem that needs to be identified.

How you address the issue is quite dependent on the nature of the condition. There are three categories of muscle trauma:

- Nonarticulate issues: Sprains and strains
- Articulate issues
- Myopathies

Nonarticulate Issues: Sprains and Strains

Generally the least serious forms of muscle traumas appear as hematomas, which are localized collections of blood, usually clotted, in a tissue or organ. Hematomas can occur almost anywhere on the body. In minor injuries, the blood is absorbed unless infection develops. Contusions (bruises) and black eyes are the most familiar forms of hematoma and will usually heal within a few days. As a good practice, we usually avoid massaging the affected area while it is healing.

Hematomas can be especially serious when they occur inside the skull, where they can place local pressure on the brain, or in instances when a person has hemophilia or a related blood-clotting disease. In these cases massage is generally contraindicated, or should involve only very light pressure.

The majority of injuries to the musculoskeletal system result in sprains and strains to the affected area, and when this happens, you become witness to the wondrous ability of muscles to repair themselves. Massage is a terrific way to encourage this process by stimulation, which brings nutrients, oxygen, and relaxation to the affected area.

Sprains

A sprain is an injury to a ligament—the strong, fibrous tissues that connect bones together. The most common function of ligaments is to hold and stabilize structures, so the most commonly injured ligaments are in the ankle, knee, and wrist. Ligaments can be injured by being stretched too far from their normal position.

The most common symptoms of a sprain are pain, swelling, and bruising of the affected joint. Symptoms will vary with the intensity of the sprain.

Strains

A strain is an injury to a muscle or tendon. Just as muscles move the skeleton, tendons are the attachment sites of muscles to the bones. When a muscle contracts it pulls on a tendon, which in turn is connected to a bone. If muscles are stretched too far, or stretched while contracting, a strain can occur. A strain is a stretching or tear of the muscle or tendon.

Strains are either the cause or symptom of a great majority of episodic pain, including headaches. Some of the main contributors to strains are stress, inadequate muscle strength, poor posture, excess body weight, and poor bending and lifting techniques.

Stress can be a major contributor to the effects of strains in two important ways. Stress causes muscles to remain in prolonged states of contraction, therefore reducing blood flow to the tissues and causing fatigue that can eventually develop into a strain. In addition, stress hormones heighten the perception of pain.

While strains can occur suddenly, for example, through exercise or accidents, more often than not they develop gradually through poor physical and mental habits.

The positive side to this equation is that lifestyle adjustments, including regular massage, exercise, and toning or using muscles in a healthy manner, can often reverse and eliminate the conditions that lead to strain and general pain in our muscles.

Treating an area of the body undergoing a strain or sprain depends on its severity. Generally speaking, once a strain or sprain has occurred and the area has swelling, one should abide by the principles of RICER: rest, ice, compression, elevation, rehabilitation.

Initially the body needs time to recover on its own. Once that phase is completed—

which takes anywhere from a few days to a few months—rehabilitation and movement are essential to full recovery, and regular Thai Yoga Massage can make an important contribution to achieving effective results.

Articulate Issues

This group refers to issues that arise at the joints, and may refer to a vast list of injuries. However, some of the more common conditions include arthritis, bursitis, tendinitis, frozen shoulder, and fibromyalgia.

Arthritis

Just about all of these conditions can be considered some form of arthritis, which literally means "joint" (from the Greek *arthro*) "inflammation" (*-itis*). There are more than one hundred different kinds of arthritis, and we will touch on a few of these.

Inflammation is one of the body's natural responses to injuries. Warning signs that inflammation is present are redness, swelling, heat, and pain. When a joint becomes inflamed, it may show any or all of these symptoms. This can prevent normal use of the joint and therefore cause the loss or function of that joint. No one knows exactly why arthritis happens, but science offers many clues.

While the triggers for inflammation remain unknown, we do understand how it manifests. Between the bones is a joint cavity, which gives the bones room to move. This cavity, or joint space between two bones, is enclosed by a capsule that's flexible, yet strong enough to protect the joint against dislocation. The inner lining of this capsule, the synovium, produces a thick fluid that lubricates and nourishes the joint. In many forms of arthritis, the synovium becomes inflamed and thickened, producing extra fluid that contains inflammatory cells. The inflamed synovium and fluid can damage the cartilage and underlying bone.

Mild Forms of Arthritis

The more mild forms of arthritis include tendinitis, bursitis, and tennis elbow. Tendinitis, as the name implies, is inflammation of a tendon. Its most common causes are overuse, ill-fitting apparel that puts abnormal tension on the tendons, and excess body weight, which can also put too much pressure on the feet and legs. Tennis elbow is a nickname for tendinitis of the elbow, as it usually occurs through playing sports. Some of the symptoms associated with tendinitis include sharp pains, tenderness, swelling, and restricted movement of the injured area.

Bursitis refers to an inflammation of the bursa, which is a fluid-filled sac that acts as a cushion between muscles, tendons, and bones.

Other Forms of Arthritis

Other types of arthritis include systemic chronic forms, such as rheumatoid arthritis; pain syndromes, such as fibromyalgia (discussed later in greater detail); and osteoarthritis.

Osteoarthritis is one of the oldest and most common forms of arthritis. Known as the "wear-and-tear" kind of arthritis, it is a chronic condition characterized by the breakdown of the joint's cartilage. The breakdown of cartilage causes the bones to rub against each other, causing stiffness, pain, and loss of movement in the joint.

Osteoarthritis most commonly occurs in the weight-bearing joints of the hips, knees, and lower back. It also affects the neck, small finger joints, base of the thumb, and big toe.

Rheumatoid arthritis is a chronic disease, mainly characterized by inflammation of the synovium of the joints. It can lead to long-term joint damage, resulting in chronic pain, loss of function, and disability.

Rheumatoid arthritis can start in any joint, but it most commonly begins in the smaller joints of the fingers, hands, and wrists. Joint involvement is usually symmetrical, meaning that if a joint hurts on the left hand, the same joint will hurt on the right hand. In general, more joint erosion indicates more severe disease activity.

As a general rule, most articulate issues can be massaged and you should see some reduction of symptoms and help with the pain. They require a gentle touch, much care, and a long-term approach. Active rheumatoid arthritis is the only articulate issue that is fully contraindicated, and you should avoid giving *or* receiving a Thai Yoga Massage if you have this condition.

Myopathies

Myopathies refer to diseases and neuromuscular disorders of the muscles in which the primary symptom is dysfunction of the muscle fiber. They are either genetic (for example, muscular dystrophy) or acquired (for example, muscle cramps). Myopathies can affect the nerves that speak to muscles, or they can affect the muscles themselves.

Muscle weakness has many causes, only some of which are related to an actual disease of the muscles. Normally, electrical signals travel from the brain through the spinal cord and into the nerves that lead to the muscles. From there, they are transmitted into the muscles, where the signals stimulate muscle tissue to contract. Along the way the nerves must be in good working order, hormones and chemicals in good supply, and the muscles must be able to accept impulses and generate a response.

Problems can occur anywhere along this route. If the brain, spinal cord, or nerves are damaged or diseased, the electrical signal may not be generated or not able to get through at a specific point. If muscles or tendons are inflamed or abnormal, they may not be able to respond properly to a nerve impulse.

Treatments for myopathies depend on the disease or condition and specific causes. Supportive and symptomatic treatment may be the only treatment available or necessary for some disorders. Treatment for other disorders may include drug therapy (for example, immunosuppressives), physical therapy, bracing to support weakened muscles, and surgery.

The prognosis for individuals with a myopathy varies. Some individuals have a normal life span and little or no disability. For others, however, the disorder may be progressive, severely disabling, life-threatening, or even fatal.

Generally Thai Yoga Massage, which helps to profoundly relax the body as well as tone muscles, is a very effective way to help relieve some of the immediate discomfort caused by myopathies.

Some of the more common groups of myopathies include:

Common muscle cramps and stiffness: This is characterized by prolonged spasms of the arms and legs.

Muscular dystrophies: There are a number of different types of muscular dystrophy. They are all inherited disorders that cause progressive muscle disease in voluntary muscles due to defects in one or more genes. The diseases are distinguished from one another by the type of symptoms seen and by the nature of the genetic abnormality causing the disorder.

Inflammatory muscle diseases: These are muscle diseases that cause inflammation of the muscles and are usually differentiated by the pattern of the onset of symptoms, as well as muscles affected. They are rare disorders and symptoms can appear suddenly or over a period of months or years. Some of the different types include dermatomyositis, polymyositis, and inclusion body myositis.

Mitochondrial myopathies: These are a group of neuromuscular diseases caused by damage to the mitochondria—small, energy-producing structures found in every cell in the body, which serve as the cells' "power plants."

OTHER CONSIDERATIONS

Now with a basic understanding of some of the ways muscle traumas present themselves, we'll take a more in-depth look at a few common ailments and some of the suggested ways you can treat them. One important thing to keep in mind is the old adage that one should always err on the side of caution. If you are ever unsure, the best strategy is to kindly refer your client to an appropriate health care professional. Furthermore, the moment itself is what truly frames your massage approach. Case studies should be used to provide more clues on how to proceed, but this is only one aspect that needs to be considered. Here are some other things to keep in mind when deciding on your massage approach:

1. What are the client's abilities and limitations? For example, can she lie on her back? Can she touch her toes?

2. What are your abilities and limitations? Is this your fourth massage of the day? Is the person a lot bigger than you are? How are you feeling?

3. How much experience does your client have with you and with Thai Yoga Massage? Is this session part of an ongoing treatment plan? Will you have to earn the trust of your client or is he ready to release to all your massage choices? Will certain stretches be conceived as too much or possibly even too proximate at this time?

❁ STRESS

In today's world, whether working as a politician, office worker, teacher, or whatever else, nobody is free from stress. Left unchecked, it is a known fact that stress can have negative effects on your health and quality of life. Stress can also be a positive force if you know how to use it, as it can help motivate you to get things done and accomplish your goals.

The concept of stress dates to the 1930s and the work of a McGill University endocrinologist named Hans Selye in identifying the body's reaction to situational pressure, otherwise known as "general adaptation syndrome." What Selye showed is that when a person is exposed to a stressful situation, the body releases up to 1,400 responses to maintain control of the situation. This initial phase is often regarded as the fight-or-flight response. The word *stress* might be new, but the response itself dates back to prehistoric times. Whether your boss is giving you a serious tongue-lashing or you are being attacked by a lion, your body reacts the same way. Heart rate speeds up, blood vessels constrict, and chemicals release into your bloodstream to strengthen and heighten your response as you prepare to defend yourself.

Once the perceived danger recedes, when you go back to your work or run away, your body usually returns to its normal phase. At least, that's what is supposed to happen. But it doesn't always work out that way. Sometimes we remain on edge after the threat has passed. We fear the lion will come back or that our livelihood is on the line, so the stress response continues. The human body has a limited number of resources and eventually, if we do not give ourselves time to recover, we can drain our immune system, which may then lead to a whole host of different illnesses. This is why stress is so often considered a leading cause of illness, from colds and body pain to more serious diseases such as cancer, heart disease, and depression.

Causes of Stress

Stress is caused by a stressor—a stressful incident or situation—that prompts your body to enter the fight-or-flight stage. From heavy exercise to sitting in traffic and obsessing, pretty much anything can cause such a response. There are many indicators to help you recognize that your body is under stress, including exhaustion, fluctuations in appetite, sweating, grinding your teeth, nervousness, and forgetfulness. The key to recognizing the signs is to pay attention to your body. If something doesn't feel quite right, most likely you are feeling the effects of stress.

When the sympathetic nervous system is constantly on the go, stress starts to have an impact on the body's functioning; for example, causing the heart rate to accelerate. The body will counter this by activating the parasympathetic system, which is in charge of relaxing us. The good news is that effective strategies and mechanisms are available to help manage and reduce your stress levels. Regular Thai Yoga Massage is among the best methods available, as shown in the case study that follows.

THAI YOGA MASSAGE TREATMENT

STRESS CASE STUDY

Recipient: Terrell Odom

Age: 55

Sex: Male

Height: 6'0"

Weight: 205 lbs.

Occupation: Investment banker

Presenting Issues: Stress, exhaustion

History: Works a standard fifty-five-hour week managing many valuable investment portfolios. Has been seriously affected by a recent economic downturn. Unable to eat properly, sometimes sleeps fewer than three hours a day, sometimes more than fourteen, then still has trouble getting out of bed.

Client has been in the financial industry for the past twenty years and has carved out a steady clientele and a very good living, but lately he has lost a few clients. He exercises at the gym three mornings a week and is usually able to eat whatever he wants with no problem, but lately finds he is less hungry and also constipated. This is his first Thai Yoga Massage, but he has received table massage over the years.

Massage Approach
Posture Customization

- Client is of large build, so eliminate anything too strenuous for you and use feet and knees where possible.
- This massage is less about the postures and more about helping to induce a quality of relaxation and circulation.

- Lots of sweeping should accompany postures for a greater relaxation effect.
- An extended foot and abdomen massage will help unwind stress.

Sen Lines

- Kalathari, Ittha, Pingkhala

Ayurveda

- Kapha build, vata imbalance (Issues of the nervous system and digestion point to a vata-decreasing massage.)
- Pace: Slow
- Pressure: Firm but not too strong
- Postures: Balance of spinal twists, forward bends, backbends
- Vayus (subtle energies):* Prana, Vyana, Apana
- Marma points: Gulpha, Nabhi, Sthapani, Adhipati

Contraindication

Stress and age could mean the possibility of high blood pressure. Be sure to ask this question in your interview, and if client is unsure of his blood pressure, eliminate inverted postures in which the legs are raised above the body. Postures such as the Half Plough, Butterfly, and AG (antigravitational spinal relaxation) poses may raise blood pressure temporarily.

Lifestyle Approach

Generally treat for the vata imbalance but keep in mind the kapha physique. For example, choose vata foods that are not too heavy on oils.

Yoga Routine Recommendations

- Forward bend
- Cobra
- Standing twist, such as Triangle
- Hugging knees to chest
- Five-minute relaxation

Food Recommendations

- Nurturing foods that help counter vata stress, but are not high in fats
- Stews, soups, khichuri (a traditional rice and lentil "comfort" dish)

---

*For discussion of vayus, please refer to *Thai Yoga Massage for Your Body Type.*

- Whole-grain breads
- Some fish
- Organic foods when possible

Lifestyle Recommendations

- Take more time for yourself.
- Keep good company with people who inspire you.
- Routine exercise practice: walking, yoga, swimming.
- Receive regular Thai Yoga Massage.

After Treatment

For progress to continue, it is recommended that the client return for regular Thai Yoga Massage treatments as often as once a week until stress symptoms recede, then follow-up with regular visits every three to four weeks.

A Word of Caution

While this treatment may prove to be effective, it does not replace medical advice from a doctor.

PUTTING IT ALL TOGETHER:
60-MINUTE THERAPEUTIC GENERAL STRESS MASSAGE

Posture	Book*	Page #	Notes
Sitting Postures			
Namaskar	3	70	
Palming Shoulders	3	71	
Rolling Pin	1	61	
Prayer Pose	1	70	Extended sweeping
Fish	2	99	
Counter Fish	2	101	
Amsa Pressure	2	102	
Foot Postures			
Palming Insteps	1	73	
Footfold	1	76	
Thumbing Sen on Sole	1	77	Sen Kalathari, Ittha, Pingkhala
Foot and Ankle Rotation	1	78	
Thumbing Sen on Dorsal	1	80	Gulpha marma, Sen Kalathari, Ittha, Pingkhala
Mortar and Pestle	2	107	Extended sweeping
Single Leg Postures			
Walking on Sen/Kneeing on Inner Leg	3	83–84	Sen Kalathari
Tree	1	88	
Angel Twist	1	90	
Knee to Forehead	1	92	
Hurricane Kick	1	93	
Knee Stretch	1	94	
Side Position Postures			
Palming the Arm Laterally	1	101	
Divine Neck Massage	3	109	Finish with extended sweeping
Shoulder Rotation	1	102	
Back Postures			
Sole Walk	1	107	
Back Massage	1	111	Work all sen lines and many variations that reduce thumb work to work out tension in head, neck, shoulders, and back
	2	127	
	3	120	
Pillow Cobra	1	114	Finish with extended sweeping and light chopping
Double Leg Postures			
Crescent Moon	2	133	
Hip Hop	1	122	
Thai Lute	2	137	Extended stretch and shaking the legs
Abdomen, Arm/Hand/Head Massage			
Abdomen 1 Massage	1	125	Nabhi marma, lots of repetition, work the chest and sternum
Arm/Hand/Head Massage	1	130, 135	Sthapani, Adhipati marma
Sitting Posture			
Namaskar	3	70	

*Book 1 = *Thai Yoga Massage*, Book 2 = *Thai Yoga Therapy for Your Body Type*, Book 3 = *Advanced Thai Yoga Massage*

❁ BACK PAIN

One of the more interesting things I ever read in *National Geographic* was an article on some of the compromises the human body had to make in order to be able to walk on two feet. The shifting of the hips, the curvature of the spine, the reformation of the knees, and the growth of the feet are all a marvel of evolutionary ingenuity. Yet at the same time, it is a fragile construction that requires good lifestyle choices or trouble will ensue.

There is little doubt that back pain is one of the most common ailments in North America. Experts believe that a major factor is the modern tendency to lead a sedentary lifestyle, both at work and home. Spending long stretches of time sitting in one position—often with the back not properly supported—is not good for the spine. Soft furnishings may seem appealing, but often they encourage poor posture. Back pain is less common in Asia, where many more people are accustomed to sitting on the floor, which is thought to allow the back muscles to find their own natural position.

Causes of Back Pain

It's difficult to pin down the exact cause of back pain, due to the complex nature of the spine, nerves, and muscles. Back pain is actually most often a symptom. The most common indicator is when the back muscles begin to spasm. This can occur after strenuous activity or as a reaction to repetitive strain. Other causes of back pain include arthritis, fractures, and infections. In many cases, experts believe back pain is a manifestation of emotional stress, rather than a result of physical misuse.

The lower—or lumbar—region of the back is particularly prone to injury, for at least two good reasons: The low back bears the weight of the entire upper body, and it twists and bends more than other parts. And everyday activities, such as walking in thick soles or high heels, can cause shock waves of strain up the heel, knees, and legs before it is eventually felt in the back.

In analyzing the way Thai Yoga Massage works, one could make the argument that it was practically invented to help people release lower back pain and tension. With a full body treatment that focuses on leg work, releasing energy blockages, chopping, twisting, and massaging, it is often just what the doctor ordered. At the same time, it takes a skilled practitioner to apply these amazing tools with great care and awareness while working this particularly sensitive area of discomfort that may have been years in developing.

THAI YOGA MASSAGE TREATMENT

BACK PAIN CASE STUDY

Recipient: Earl Jones

Age: 43

Sex: Male

Height: 5'10"

Weight: 185 lbs.

Occupation: Bus driver

Presenting Issues: Nagging lower back pain, sore right knee

History: Drives a regular seven-hour route between Toronto and Montreal four times a week. Back pain began to surface four years ago. Throbbing pain comes and goes throughout the day. Is aware of the pain but it's more a nuisance than "real pain." Within the past two weeks it has gotten worse and the client is hoping the massage can help relieve the pain. The knee pain is new, not attributed to any particular activity, and he just woke up with it a couple of days ago.

Client has been a bus driver for thirteen years and enjoys the steady pay. His only form of exercise is walking to and from work. He enjoys watching TV to relax most evenings, or spending time with his wife and two children. He eats three meals a day and is a meat and potatoes man, but is switching more and more to chicken and fish. He drinks three to five cups of coffee a day and sleeps seven hours a night. He has occasional heartburn but overall good digestion. Generally feels good except for the sore back. He heard about Thai Yoga Massage from a friend who has had excellent results, and this is his first treatment.

Massage Approach
Posture Customization

- Client is of medium build; his size relative to yours should be taken into consideration and any postures that could be a strain for you should be eliminated.
- Focus on movements to help circulate energy, move the trunk, and relax the back and hips, including the Half Plough, Cobra, Mini AG, Angel Twist, Pigeon Stretch, and North/South Stretches, such as extended shaking of the legs and a Long Stretch.

- Eliminate the sitting positions, since he sits for long periods of time every day, and give the back massage from the side, as that would be more comfortable for him than lying prone.

Sen Lines

- Kalathari, Ittha, Pingkhala, Thawari, Sahatsarangsi

Ayurveda

- Kapha/pitta build, pitta imbalance
- Pace: Medium
- Pressure: Firm but not too strong
- Postures: Balance gentle spinal twists with articulations and forward bends
- Vayus: Vyana, Samana
- Marma points: Kukundara, Janu, Gulpha, Basti Nabhi

Contraindication

If you choose to massage the back while the recipient is lying prone, avoid using Sanuk posture, because there is a danger of aggravating the lower back when lifting over and sliding into position. Nevertheless, a good palming and elbowing on the buttocks can be very relieving.

Lifestyle Approach

Since the client sits in the same position and uses the same motions over and over again, all remediation should be geared toward stimulation and movement.

Yoga Routine Recommendations

- Cat stretch
- Side-lying twist
- Forward bend
- Hugging knees to chest
- Three-minute relaxation

Food Recommendations

- Encourage the switch to more chicken and fish. The body needs movement to assist proper digestion, and heavy meats tax the system.
- Try to reduce coffee consumption and replace with more pitta friendly fruits (such as apples, bananas, and berries) and fruit juices.

PUTTING IT ALL TOGETHER:
60-MINUTE THERAPEUTIC BACK MASSAGE

Posture	Book*	Page #	Notes
Sitting Posture			
Namaskar	3	70	
Foot Postures			
Palming Insteps	1	73	
Foot Fold	1	76	
Foot and Ankle Rotation	1	78	
Foot Spinal Twist	1	79	
Thumbing Sen on Sole	1	77	Sen Kalathari, Ittha, Pingkhala
Thumbing Sen on Dorsal	1	80	Sen Kalathari, Ittha, Pingkhala
Milk the Cow	1	82	
Single Leg Postures			
Palming/Thumbing Sen	1	84	Sen Kalathari, Thawari, Sahatsarangsi
Helicopter	1	97	
Tree	1	88	
High Heel	1	89	Including extended calf massage
Angel Twist	1	90	
Pigeon Stretch	3	88	
Double Foot Hurricane	3	92	
Knee Stretch	1	94	
Uranus	1	95	Size permitting
Knee to Forehead	1	92	
Helicopter	1	97	Extended light chopping and sweeping
Side Position Postures			
Dragon Twist	1	100	Gradual approach
Kneeling Leg Fold	3	103	
Back Walk	3	104	Access Janu marma with foot behind the knee
Divine Neck Massage	3	109	Finish with extended sweeping
Double Leg Postures			
Half Plough	1	118	
Tortoise	2	135	One leg at a time
Half Mini AG	3	86	
Hip Hop	1	122	
Thai Lute	2	137	Extended stretch and shaking the legs
Long Stretch	1	117	
Abdomen Massage			
Abdomen 1 Massage	1	125	Focus on Samana Vayu
Sitting Posture			
Namaskar	3	70	

*Book 1 = *Thai Yoga Massage*, Book 2 = *Thai Yoga Therapy for Your Body Type*, Book 3 = *Advanced Thai Yoga Massage*

Lifestyle Recommendations

- Keep good company with people who inspire you.
- Routine exercise practice: Pilates, yoga, and swimming; being active without putting a strain on the back.
- Be mindful of body position in all daily activities—standing, sitting, lifting, sleeping—so as not to aggravate the situation. (For instance, lift objects by squatting with a straight back and standing up slowly rather than bending over and lifting with the back.)
- If the pain continues, visit a doctor and osteopath for further examination.

After Treatment

For progress to continue, it is recommended that the client return for regular Thai Yoga Massage treatments as often as once a week until the stress recedes, then follow-up with regular visits every three to four weeks.

A Word of Caution

While this treatment may prove to be effective, it does not replace medical advice from a doctor.

❁ STIFF NECK AND SORE SHOULDERS

Quite possibly, the most common of common ailments is stiffness, soreness, and pain in the shoulder and neck regions. We never fail to elicit laughter in class when we mention the good possibility of finding beans, marbles, or the occasional golf ball–sized tension lumps on people's shoulders and neck. These contracted knots speak to the direct connection between mind and body, demonstrating how mental and emotional stress can have an impact on the body if proper care isn't taken.

The brain can be seen as the body's power station, and the spinal cord is like the primary power lines that then branch out to secondary channels throughout the body. Therefore, tension and energy blockage in the neck and shoulders can restrict the health and vitality of the body. The closer the blockage to the power station, the more vulnerable one is to a host of pain and illnesses, and when tension is released there, all of the bodily systems tend to operate more smoothly and efficiently.

Stiffness in the neck is usually accompanied by soreness in the shoulder muscles, most notably the trapezius, deltoid, and deeper rhomboid muscles. It is difficult to say if one causes the other, but almost everyone at some point in life will feel the effects of a stiff neck and sore shoulders, and any thorough massage treatment will work the whole neck and shoulder area.

Causes of Stiff Neck and Sore Shoulders

The muscles and bones of the neck have to support the weight of the head and every turn the head makes. Neck pain may come from any element in the structure of the neck, including the vertebrae and muscles of the upper back, the blood vessels of the neck, or lymph nodes in the neck.

Many types of injuries or illnesses can result in a stiff neck, including sleeping in a window draft, holding the telephone awkwardly, or even worn shock absorbers in a car. Similarly, stiff shoulders can result from hundreds of different possibilities caused by repetitive strain, unconscious actions, and allowing conditions to continue over time. Conditions may include poor posture, work overload, or the emotional feelings of "carrying the weight of the world on your shoulders."

In most cases the muscles are overworked, which leads the muscles to spasm; that is, the brain sends signals for the muscles to work or contract, which leads over time to knots that can become progressively pronounced and painful.

Thai Yoga Massage treatment and stretching can often help to decrease the knots, release spasms in the muscles, and give better mobility to this area, in both short- and long-term regular treatments.

THAI YOGA MASSAGE TREATMENT

STIFF NECK AND SORE SHOULDERS CASE STUDY

Recipient: Krystal Chang

Age: 35

Sex: Female

Height: 5'2"

Weight: 110 lbs.

Occupation: Marketing consultant

Presenting Issues: Chronic neck and shoulder pain, numbness in right arm

History: Dedicated, hard-working entrepreneur who started her own business eight years ago. Works at least forty-five hours a week and rarely takes a vacation. Many hours are spent in front of the computer, talking on the phone, and multitasking, as well as traveling and meeting with clients. She feels as though the wear and tear and stress of it all is catching up to her, and her neck pain can sometimes last up to a week at a time. Usually feels soreness in her shoulders throughout the day. Currently has stiffness in her neck and general shoulder tension but can move her head with some discomfort. The arm numbness has been acting up over the past couple of months and she believes it is all related.

Client exercises two or three times a week with a combination of weight training, aerobics, and jogging. Married, with two elementary school children, whom she adores. Eats a moderately vegetarian and mostly organic diet. She knows she works hard, but has plenty of stamina, has created a successful business, and is very excited about her future prospects.

Massage Approach
Posture Customization

- Postures should include deep work on the neck and shoulders at various points in the massage, and then give some time to relax before returning to the area of attention.

- Spend an extended amount of time in sitting positions to get right to the heart of the matter, primarily through Ultimate Rolling Pin. Balance it up with twists and a forward bend to relax the whole upper body.
- In this case a full-body massage is advised in order to work the sen lines in their entirety and because of the ripple effects of balancing the energy throughout the central nervous system.

Sen Lines

- Kalathari, Ittha, Pingkhala, Thawari, Sahatsarangsi

Ayurveda

- Vata-pitta build, vata imbalance
- Pace: Slow
- Pressure: Firm, but not too vigorous
- Postures: Articulations, twists, and movements that encourage circulation and movements of the spine
- Vayus: Vyana, Apana, Prana
- Marma points: Amsa, Krikatika, Brihati, Kurpara

Contraindication

Special care should be taken to protect and respect the cervical spine and put no strain on the neck. Do not crack the neck or apply sudden or jerky movements, and avoid stretches where the neck may hang or constrict, such as the Metta Hug, Dead Man Twist, Tea Kettle Twists, and Lunar Stretch.

Lifestyle Approach

Since the client has repetitive motions she must use in her work, special care should be taken to gently correct the way she uses her body.

Yoga Routine Recommendations

- Forward bend
- Side-lying twist
- Hugging knees to chest
- Five-minute relaxation

Food Recommendations

The practitioner should use the Ayurvedic Food Guidelines table in *Thai Yoga Therapy for Your Body Type* (pages 173–76). Remember to make recommendations from a point of view of abundance. There are many foods that can be eaten regularly and some that are more of a treat. Review the lists with the client and add foods that are soothing to vata. It is best to recommend a few attainable changes at a time.

Lifestyle Recommendations

- Keep good company with people who inspire you.
- Routine exercise practice: yoga, neck, and shoulder strengthening exercises.
- Receive regular Thai Yoga Massage.
- Assess office habits and sleeping conditions for better posture.
- If the pain continues, visit a doctor and osteopath for further examination.

After Treatment

For progress to continue, it is recommended that the client return for regular Thai Yoga Massage treatments as often as once a week until the stress recedes, then follow-up with regular visits every three to four weeks.

A Word of Caution

While this treatment may prove to be effective, it does not replace medical advice from a doctor.

PUTTING IT ALL TOGETHER:
60-MINUTE THERAPEUTIC SHOULDER AND NECK MASSAGE

Posture	Book*	Page #	Notes
Sitting Postures			
Namaskar	3	70	
Palming Shoulders	3	71	
Ultimate Rolling Pin	3	73	Massaging all parts of neck and shoulders
Shakti Twist	2	93	
Shoulder Squeeze	3	78	
Neck Massage	1	65	
Jade Pillow	1	66	
Prayer Pose	1	70	
Fish	2	99	Support the neck
Counter Fish	2	101	Very gently
Amsa Pressure	2	102	
Foot Postures			
Thumbing Sen on Sole	1	77	Sen Kalathari, Ittha, Pingkhala, Thawari, Sahatsarangsi
Thumbing Sen on Dorsal	1	80	Sen Kalathari, Ittha, Pingkhala, Thawari, Sahatsarangsi
Single Leg Postures			
Palming/Thumbing Sen	1	84	Sen Kalathari, Thawari, Sahatsarangsi
Helicopter	1	97	
Tree	1	88	
Nataraj	2	114	
Side Kick	1	91	
Diva Twist	1	98	
Side Position Postures			
Shoulder Rotation	1	102	
Divine Neck Massage	3		Krikatika marma, finish with extended sweeping
Back Postures			
Back Massage	1	111	Brihati, Amsa, Krikatika marma, shoulder stretch, all sen lines
	3	120	
Pillow Cobra	1	114	
Double Leg Postures			
Half Plough	1	118	
Butterfly	1	120	
Hip Hop	1	122	
Thai Lute	2	137	Extended stretch and shaking the legs
Long Stretch	1	117	
Abdomen, Arm/Hand/Head Massage			
Opening the Chest	2	143	Sweep, circle sternum
Arm-Hand Massage	1	130	Kurpara marma
Head Massage	1	135	Include jade pillow and shoulder massage
Sitting Posture			
Namaskar	3	70	

*Book 1 = *Thai Yoga Massage*, Book 2 = *Thai Yoga Therapy for Your Body Type*, Book 3 = *Advanced Thai Yoga Massage*

❀ TIRED ARMS AND HANDS

One of the prime factors that separates humans from our brothers and sisters in the animal kingdom is the incredible functionality of our arms and hands. With the power to punch through a wood board and the precision to thread a needle, there is no end to our capacity to create, build, and make our mark in the world. However, we tend to take this remarkable ability for granted, expecting that our arms and hands will respond to our needs forever and never wear out from over- or misuse. As a consequence, there are a plethora of ailments that affect both. Carpal tunnel syndrome, tendinitis, arthritis, and bursitis are just some of the more common afflictions.

As marvelous a creation as our arms and hands are, we need to recognize that they can certainly tire out, and they do so far more often than we realize. In fact, if we recognize that and treat them to a little rest and relaxation on a regular basis, many of the problems that creep up later in life are easily preventable.

Causes of Tired Arms and Hands

People use their hands and arms in so many ways throughout the day that it is difficult to pinpoint precise reasons why they get tired. Some of the more obvious reasons include repetitive activities, the most prevalent these days being typing at a computer and driving a car. But problems can occur in both sedentary and active lifestyles. If you are a painter, exercise regularly in a gym, drive regularly for a living, work in an office, play tennis, chop tons of vegetables, lift heavy items, or a myriad of other daily activities, you probably tire out your arms and hands on a regular basis. Many of the technique applications used in Thai Yoga Massage are specifically designed to keep therapists from tiring their arms and hands.

If you feel numbness, shooting pain, or any of a number of other indicators, you already have a problem and should seek attention before it becomes worse. Better yet is to realize that you use your arms and hands in thousands of different ways every day, so take a little time to rest and rehabilitate them and they will thank you.

Thai Yoga Massage, with its articulations, stretching, and massage, is a great way to help remedy tired arms and hands. Therefore, let this be a reminder to all practitioners that including this work in every massage is essential for maintaining the optimal well-being of your clients for the long term.

THAI YOGA MASSAGE TREATMENT

TIRED ARMS AND HANDS CASE STUDY

Recipient: Karl Buettner

Age: 38

Sex: Male

Height: 5'8"

Weight: 160 lbs.

Occupation: Massage therapist

Presenting Issues: Tired arms and hands, shoulder tension

History: A massage therapist for the past ten years giving fifteen to twenty massages per week. Rarely receives massage and has noticed occasional shooting pain in his right elbow and wrist. Determined to nip it in the bud before the problem progresses. Also feels regular tension in his shoulders from his work. Spends another twenty hours a week doing volunteer work. Has always wanted to receive more massage but hasn't taken the time.

Erratic schedule, mostly does volunteer work in the morning and massage work during the late afternoon and evenings, so usually has a late dinner and difficulty falling asleep before 1:30 a.m.

Massage Approach

Posture Customization

- ◆ Focus is to massage and stretch out the arms, hands, and shoulders at various points throughout the massage.
- ◆ Tired arms and hands can also reflect blockages in the neck and back, so they should also receive a good workout.
- ◆ Lots of moderate chopping followed by calming sweeping should accompany postures.

Sen Lines

- ◆ Kalathari for the whole body, Ittha, Pingkhala, Thawari, Sahatsarangsi in the upper body

Ayurveda

- Pitta build, pitta imbalance (pitta-decreasing massage)
- Pace: Medium
- Pressure: Firm, but not too strong
- Postures: Mostly spinal twists, traction, articulation, with some forward bends
- Vayus: Prana, Vyana, Apana
- Marma points: Amsa, Kurpara, Kshipra

Contraindication

Vyana Vayu, which has heating qualities, will be engaged here to stimulate circulation along the arms and hands. Balance this out with gentle sweeping and a calming end to your massage to soothe the fiery pitta nature. A lot of chronic tiredness is due to bad body postures, hyperextending the arms and wrists, and excessive use of thumbs.

Lifestyle Approach
Yoga Routine Recommendations

- Forward bend
- Standing spinal twist
- Circles with arms and wrists
- Self-hand massage
- Five-minute relaxation

Food Recommendations

- If possible, eat before the last massage of the day.
- Raw foods
- Cool grains, such as basmati rice and whole wheat
- Some protein, including nuts and seeds throughout the day to maintain energy through a busy schedule
- Organic foods when possible

Lifestyle Recommendations

- Keep good company with people who inspire you.
- Get to sleep earlier.
- Routine exercise practice: walking, yoga, swimming.
- Receive regular Thai Yoga Massage.

PUTTING IT ALL TOGETHER:
60-MINUTE THERAPEUTIC TIRED ARMS AND HANDS MASSAGE

Posture	Book*	Page #	Notes
Sitting Postures			
Namaskar	3	70	
Palming Shoulders	3	71	
Ultimate Rolling Pin	3	73	
Cow Face 1	1	62	
Cow Face 2	1	64	
Shiva Twist	2	92	
Shakti Twist	2	93	
Butterfly Knee	2	90	
Row Boat	1	69	
Prayer Pose	1	70	Extended chopping
Amsa Pressure	2	102	
Foot Postures			
Thumbing Sen on Sole	1	77	Sen Kalathari
Thumbing Sen on Dorsal	1	80	Gulpha marma, Sen Kalathari
Single Leg Postures			
Walking on Sen/Kneeing on Inner Leg	3	83–84	Sen Kalathari
Tree	1	88	
Nataraj	2	114	
Knee to Forehead	1	92	
Diva Twist	1	98	
Side Position Postures			
Shoulder Rotation	1	102	
Side Arm Extension	3	107	
Shoulder Swing	3	108	
Devil Stretch	1	103	
Divine Neck Massage	3	109	Finish with extended sweeping
Back Postures			
Back Massage	1	111	Work Sen Kalathari, Ittha, Pingkhala,
	2	127	Thawari, Sahatsarangsi and add
	3	120	variations that reduce thumb work to work out tension in shoulders and arms
Shoulder Stretch	3	119	
Pillow Cobra	1	114	Finish with extended sweeping and light chopping
Arm/Hand/Head Massage			
Arm/Hand/Head massage	1	130, 135	Work Sen Kalathari, Ittha, Pingkhala, Thawari, Sahatsarangsi, Kurpara, Kshipra marma, extended hand massage
Sitting Posture			
Namaskar	3	70	

*Book 1 = *Thai Yoga Massage*, Book 2 = *Thai Yoga Therapy for Your Body Type*, Book 3 = *Advanced Thai Yoga Massage*

After Treatment

To ensure long-term continuity in the profession, client should find other parts of the body to use instead of thumbs: elbows, knuckles, side of the hand, forearm, and fists. Mix it up and exercise more of the body. The client should return for regular weekly treatments; also encourage more self-massage using either tennis balls or his own hands.

A Word of Caution

While this treatment may prove to be effective, it does not replace medical advice from a doctor.

❁ TENSION HEADACHES

My teacher Asokananda is famous for his successful treatments of headaches. We joke that he works you so hard that you forget about your headache. Obviously his reputation precedes his treatment.

There are many different kinds of headaches and Western science continues to argue about their exact cause, but there is no debate for someone experiencing the effects. The most frequent kind of headache is regularly referred to as a "tension headache" or even a "stress headache." Tension headaches generally involve a dull pain or discomfort in the head, scalp, or neck, usually associated with muscle tightness in these areas. They may occur at any age, but are most common in adults and adolescents. If a headache occurs two or more times weekly for several months or for more than half a month, the condition is considered chronic.

Causes of Tension Headaches

Although there is debate as to whether muscle contractions are a cause or symptom of tension, it's generally accepted that stress not properly managed is a primary contributor to tension headaches. Furthermore, any activity that causes you to hold your head in one position for a long time without moving can cause a headache. Such activities include use of computers, prolonged talking on the phone, fine work with the hands, or even sleeping in an awkward position.

Tension headaches usually begin slowly and gradually. They often start in the middle of the day and can sometimes be more painful than migraine headaches.

I have seen many people reduce or eliminate tension headaches from their lives with the help of Thai Yoga Massage, along with overall lifestyle changes. The combination of working marma points, energy lines, and postures makes for a powerful potion to help banish those headaches.

THAI YOGA MASSAGE TREATMENT

TENSION HEADACHE CASE STUDY

Recipient: Mary St. Claire

Age: 43

Sex: Female

Height: 5'5"

Weight: 125 lbs.

Occupation: Restaurant manager

Presenting Issues: Repeated tension headaches, sore shoulders, tired feet

History: Has been working in restaurants for the past fifteen years. In charge of a very busy place, and many hours are spent on her feet carrying dishes and managing a staff of ten. Began getting headaches once or twice a month about two years ago. Headaches usually start at the back of her head and spread to the whole head. They tend to last for three to four hours.

When not working, helps care for her two teenage boys, spends time with her husband, enjoys cooking, watches TV. Tends to eat a lot of rich food, doesn't exercise outside of her work.

Massage Approach

Posture Customization

- Headaches could be related to the body being overworked, so a good amount of time should be spent massaging both the lower and upper parts.
- Headaches in a woman this age could also be due to the hormonal changes of perimenopause. The massage should focus on transmitting an energy of calm compassion and an understanding of this natural process.
- It is great to follow up the massage work of Ultimate Rolling Pin with postures for the shoulders and neck, such as Water Pump, Shiva Twist, and Shakti Twist to encourage movement and to help break up tension.
- To encourage a shift of the energy away from the head and down the body, end the massage by resting the client's back and head at an incline on a floor chair (such as a BackJack) or on a prop such as a pillow or bolster.

Sen Lines

- Thawari, Sahatsarangsi, Ulangka, Lawusang

Ayurveda

- Vata build, vata imbalance
- Pace: Slow
- Pressure: Light
- Postures: Lots of articulations along with twists, forward and backward bends
- Vayus: Apana, Vyana, Prana
- Marma points: Amsa, Krikatika, Gulpha, Janu, Kshipra, Shanka, Vidhura, Sthapani, Adhipati

Contraindication

In Thailand it might be okay to scare away a headache with intense pressure, but in the West, take care to keep the pressure lighter, as there can be a tendency to have a headache the following day when the massage is too strong or long, especially if the client isn't in good physical shape. Furthermore, it is contraindicated to work on someone while she is experiencing a headache.

Lifestyle Approach
Yoga Routine Recommendations

- Single leg raise
- Side-lying twist
- Cat stretch
- Ankle clasp
- Hugging knees to chest
- Five-minute relaxation

Food Recommendations

- Her active lifestyle encourages hearty foods and extra protein, as well as some sweet treats.
- Stews, soups, khichuri
- Whole-grain breads
- Some fish
- Organic foods when possible

Lifestyle Recommendations

- Keep good company with people who inspire you.
- Take more time for yourself.
- Routine exercise practice: yoga, walks in the park.
- Receive regular Thai Yoga Massage.
- Further assess working, home, and sleep conditions; change lighting, spend less time on feet, improve posture and sleep.
- If the headaches continue, recommend visiting a doctor and osteopath for further examination.

After Treatment

For progress to continue, it is recommended that the client return for regular Thai Yoga Massage treatments as often as once a week until the headaches diminish, then follow-up with regular visits every three to four weeks.

A Word of Caution

While this treatment may prove to be effective, it does not replace medical advice from a doctor.

PUTTING IT ALL TOGETHER:
60-MINUTE THERAPEUTIC MASSAGE FOR HEADACHES

Posture	Book*	Page #	Notes
Sitting Postures			
Namaskar	3	70	
Palming Shoulders	3	71	
Ultimate Rolling Pin	3	73	Massaging all parts of neck and shoulders
Shiva Twist	2	92	
Shakti Twist	2	93	
Jade Pillow	1	66	Working Krikatika marma
Row Boat	1	69	
Prayer Pose	1	70	Extended sweeping and light chopping
Amsa Pressure	2	102	
Foot Postures			
Plantarflexion	1	74	
Dorsiflexion	1	75	
Foot and Ankle Rotation	1	78	
Foot Spinal Twist	1	79	Gulpha marma
Mortar and Pestle	2	107	
Shoe Polish	2	108	
Single Leg Postures			
Palming/Thumbing Sen	1	84	Sen Thawari, Sahatsarangsi
Helicopter	1	97	
Nataraj	2	114	
Stringing Bow	2	115	
Single Leg Extension: palming	3	96	Extended light chopping and sweeping
Apana Release	2	117	
Side Position Postures			
Dragon Twist	1	100	
Shoulder rotation	1	102	
Divine Neck Massage	3	109	Krikatika marma finish with extended sweeping
Back Postures			
Sole Roll	2	123	Head supported with bolsters, roll on calves
Janu Pump	2	124	
Sanuk	1	109	
Back Massage	1	111	Work sen lines, shoulder stretch,
	2	127	finish with extended sweeping and
	3	120	light chopping
Double Leg Postures			
Half Plough	1	118	
Hip Hop	1	122	
Thai Lute	2	137	Extended stretch and shaking the legs
Abdomen, Arm/Hand/Head Massage			
Abdomen 1 Massage	1	125	Sweep, circle sternum
Arm, Hand Massage	1	130	Kshipra marma
Head Massage	2	147	Include all marma points at head
Sitting Posture			
Namaskar	3	70	

*Book 1 = *Thai Yoga Massage*, Book 2 = *Thai Yoga Therapy for Your Body Type*, Book 3 = *Advanced Thai Yoga Massage*

✿ CONSTIPATION

At the Lahu hill-tribe village in northern Thailand, where my teacher Asokananda and I used to conduct retreats for Thai Yoga Massage and yoga, we would see students from all over the world, with the majority coming from the West. My teacher and I were on the opposite end of the spectrum from them in our culture and habits, especially regarding food and hygiene. The diet throughout the twelve-day retreat was basically sticky rice and Lahu chilies. There were only two ways to go with this fare: either you were constipated or you had exceptionally good bowel movements. With many years of experience under our belts, we are proud to say we often had great success in treating constipation with massage and a subsidized diet of passion fruit and papaya (including the seeds), as well as yoga exercise. In the Lahu village, you were guaranteed a good bowel movement after that.

You do not need to have a bowel movement every day in order to be considered regular. A "normal" frequency of bowel movements varies widely, from three a day to three a week. What's normal for you may not be normal for someone else. In general, though, you're probably constipated if you pass hard, dry stools fewer than three times a week. In some cases, you may also feel bloated or sluggish or experience discomfort or pain.

Causes of Constipation

Normally, the waste products of digestion are propelled through your intestines by muscle contractions. In the large intestine, most of the water and salt in this mixture is reabsorbed because these elements are essential for many of your body's functions. If too much water is absorbed or if the waste moves too slowly, you can become constipated.

A number of factors can cause intestinal slowdown, including inadequate fluid intake, low-fiber diet, inattention to bowel habits, age, lack of physical activity, depression, pregnancy, illness, and even stress.

Many medications, including those used to treat high blood pressure and depression, can also cause constipation. The same is true of many narcotics. And frequent use of laxatives often aggravates and may even eventually cause constipation. In rare cases, constipation may signal a more serious medical condition.

Thai Yoga Massage is particularly effective in treating constipation because you move people—and bowels—like nobody's business! This is the only massage that twists, bends, and massages your abdomen into shape.

THAI YOGA MASSAGE TREATMENT

CONSTIPATION CASE STUDY

Recipient: Gita Lama

Age: 63

Sex: Female

Height: 5'4"

Weight: 120 lbs.

Occupation: Filmmaker

Presenting Issues: Constipation

History: Has been working as a documentary filmmaker for thirty-five years. Travels frequently for work and pleasure and enjoys eating fine, rich foods. Her lifestyle makes it difficult to cook and she generally eats in restaurants. Usually feels constipated after traveling and has just returned from two weeks of filming on location in London. This is her first Thai Yoga Massage.

Massage Approach

Posture Customization

- Client is of small build, so be aware of using too much pressure.
- This massage will use postures, energy lines, and Ayurveda to stimulate digestion.
- Postures that focus on the lower back and abdomen and twists that promote an internal massage are all great ways to target constipation.
- Also think of leg postures that push toward the bowels, such as drawn out circles in Helicopter and extended hold in Knee to Shoulder.
- Work the right side, then the left side of the body so as to move in the same direction as digestion.

Sen Lines

- Ittha, Pingkhala

Ayurveda

- Vata build, vata imbalance (vata-decreasing massage)
- Pace: Slow

- Pressure: Gentle
- Postures: Spinal twists, forward bends, backbends, large circles, and articulation of legs
- Vayus: Samana, Apana, Vyana
- Marma points: Gulpha, Kukundara, Brihati

Contraindication

Be aware of pain accompanying constipation. In these cases eliminate prone parts of the massage and proceed with an extended side-lying massage.

Lifestyle Approach
Yoga Routine Recommendations

- Abdominal churning exercise, for example, *nauli,* a yogic exercise for cleansing the digestive organs
- Forward bend
- Cobra
- Lying-down twist
- Hugging knees to chest
- Five-minute relaxation

Food Recommendations

- Avoid low-fiber or processed foods
- Minimal salt and oil, even when eating in restaurants
- Plenty of raw or simply cooked vegetables that are high in fiber
- Whole-grain breads
- Some fish
- Prune juice and lots of water
- Organic foods when possible

Lifestyle Recommendations

- Keep good company with people who inspire you.
- Routine exercise practice: walking, yoga, swimming.
- Receive regular Thai Yoga Massage.

PUTTING IT ALL TOGETHER:
60-MINUTE THERAPEUTIC CONSTIPATION MASSAGE

Posture	Book*	Page #	Notes
Sitting Posture			
Namaskar	3	70	
Foot Postures			
Foot and Ankle Rotation	1	78	Gulpha marma extended hold
Foot Spinal Twist	1	79	
Toe Arc	2	106	
Milk the Cow	1	82	Extended sweeping
Single Leg Postures			
Helicopter	1	97	Extra rotations
Tree	1	88	
Nataraj	2	114	
Stringing Bow	2	115	
Knee to Forehead	1	92	Hold for extended time
Hugging Tree	2	116	
Apana Release	2	117	
Hip Swing	3	99	
Side Position Postures			
Dragon Twist	1	100	
Back Walk	3	104	
Standing Side Arc	1	105	
Kneeling Leg Fold	3	103	
Abdomen Massage			
Abdomen Massage I	1	125	Use wave, rolling pin, substantial Sun and Moon stroke, putting more emphasis at the descending colon
Back Postures			
Thunderbolt	1	108	
Sanuk	1	109	
Locust	1	110	
Back Massage	1	111	Kukundara marma, extra focus on lower back
Pillow Cobra	1	114	Direct breathing toward internal organs
Double Leg Postures			
Yoke	1	119	
Thai Lute	2	137	Extended stretch and shaking the legs
Sitting Posture			
Namaskar	3	70	Sweep the whole body, finish with a moment of silence at the abdomen

*Book 1 = *Thai Yoga Massage*, Book 2 = *Thai Yoga Therapy for Your Body Type*, Book 3 = *Advanced Thai Yoga Massage*

After Treatment

To encourage a healthy bowel movement, drink a lot of water and try to eat soon after the massage while the system is activated. Return for weekly treatments until the system regulates, and then every four weeks.

A Word of Caution

While this treatment may prove to be effective, it does not replace medical advice from a doctor.

❁ FIBROMYALGIA

A story that comes up again and again about fibromyalgia is that a client reports that she hurts all over, frequently feels exhausted, and is often depressed. It's a triple dose of bad news, but even after numerous tests, the doctor can't seem to find anything wrong. Yet these feelings won't go away.

Fibromyalgia is a chronic and often debilitating condition characterized by fatigue; widespread pain in muscles, ligaments, and tendons; and multiple tender (trigger) points—places on the body where slight pressure causes tremendous pain.

Causes of Fibromyalgia

The specific cause of fibromyalgia is unknown. However, doctors believe a number of factors may contribute. These factors include:

- *Chemical changes in the brain.* Some people with fibromyalgia appear to have alterations in the regulation of certain brain-chemical neurotransmitters. This may be particularly true of serotonin, which is also commonly linked to depression; and substance P, a brain chemical associated with pain, stress, anxiety, and depression.
- *Sleep disturbances.* Some researchers theorize that disturbed sleep patterns may be a cause, rather than just a symptom of fibromyalgia.
- *Injury.* An injury or trauma, particularly in the upper spinal region, may trigger the development of fibromyalgia in some people. An injury may affect the central nervous system and trigger fibromyalgia.
- *Stress and hormonal changes.* These also may be possible causes, although there is no exact scientific link.

Although the symptoms will probably never disappear completely, it may be reassuring to know that fibromyalgia isn't progressive, crippling, or life-threatening. Treatments and self-care steps can improve symptoms and general health. We have had tremendous success in helping clients improve their quality of life through regular Thai Yoga Massage treatments, as the combination of metta touch, sweeping, gentle movements, and energy line massage gets right to the heart of the problem.

THAI YOGA MASSAGE TREATMENT

FIBROMYALGIA CASE STUDY

Recipient: Jeanette St. Louis

Age: 51

Sex: Female

Height: 5'0"

Weight: 150 lbs.

Occupation: Office assistant

Presenting Issues: Fibromyalgia, stress, tiredness

History: Works a forty-hour week as an office assistant in a law firm. Recently divorced after fifteen years of marriage. Sleeps only about five hours of interrupted sleep a night. Has become very sensitive to touch in her joints, back, and legs.

Eats just one large meal a day, at night; takes supplements and snacks during the day.

Massage Approach

Posture Customization

- Eliminate any strong postures and maintain a very soft nurturing touch.
- Focus on relaxation, metta, and circulating energy around the body.
- Lots of sweeping should accompany postures for a greater relaxation effect.
- Deep relaxation usually reduces the pain symptoms of fibromyalgia.

Sen Lines

- Kalathari, Ittha, Pingkhala

Ayurveda

- Kapha build, vata imbalance (Issues of body pain relate to the nervous system, therefore, this is a vata-decreasing massage.)
- Pace: Slow
- Pressure: Soft
- Postures: Balance of spinal twists, forward bends, backbends

- Vayus: Prana, Vyana
- Marma points: Gulpha, Nabhi, Sthapani, Adhipati

Contraindication

Before beginning the treatment it is very important to know the location of any points of pain. Follow the edict that "less is more" and ask for feedback regularly throughout the massage. Make sure to keep the pressure very light and focus more on palming than thumbing. Be aware that overworking an area could potentially cause pain. If that should happen, work away from that specific location.

Lifestyle Approach

Generally treat for vata imbalance but keep in mind the kapha physique. For example, choose vata foods that are not too heavy in oils.

Yoga Routine Recommendations

- Long stretch
- Cat stretch
- Lying twist
- Hugging knees to chest
- Five-minute relaxation

Food Recommendations

- Nurturing foods that help counter vata imbalances, but not high in fats
- Stews, soups, khichuri
- Whole-grain breads
- Some fish
- Organic foods when possible

Lifestyle Recommendations

- Take more time for yourself.
- Keep good company with people who inspire you.
- Routine exercise practice: walking, yoga, swimming.
- Receive regular Thai Yoga Massage.

PUTTING IT ALL TOGETHER:
60-MINUTE THERAPEUTIC FIBROMYALGIA MASSAGE

Posture	Book*	Page #	Notes
Sitting Posture			
Namaskar	3	70	
Foot Postures			
Palming Insteps	1	73	
Thumbing Sen on Sole	1	77	
Foot and Ankle Rotation	1	78	
Shoe Polish	2	108	Gulpha marma, Sen Kalathari, Ittha, Pingkhala
Toe Dance	2	109	Extended sweeping
Single Leg Postures			
Palming Sen	1	84	Sen Kalathari
Helicopter	1	97	Extra rotations
Tree	1	88	
Angel Twist	1	90	
Knee Stretch	1	94	
Snake Creeps Down	1	96	
Hip Swing	3	99	Extended sweeping
Side Position Postures			
Palming the Arm	1	101	
Shoulder Rotation	1	102	
Back Walk	3	104	
Back Postures			
Sole Roll	2	123	Palm up the back of the legs
Back Massage	1	111	Finish with extended sweeping
Double Leg Postures			
Thai Lute	2	137	
Long Stretch	1	117	
Abdomen, Arm/Hand/Head Massage			
Abdomen 1 Massage	1	125	Nabhi marma
Opening the Chest	2	143	Gentle circles and sweep the sternum
Arm/Hand/Head Massage	1	130, 135	Sthapani, Adhipati marma
Sitting Posture			
Namaskar	3	70	

*Book 1 = *Thai Yoga Massage*, Book 2 = *Thai Yoga Therapy for Your Body Type*, Book 3 = *Advanced Thai Yoga Massage*

After Treatment

Regular ongoing Thai Yoga Massage treatments are recommended, as often as once a week.

A Word of Caution

While this treatment may prove to be effective, it does not replace medical advice from a doctor.

❀ ANXIETY AND DEPRESSION

In a radio spot made by the Quebec government, a child is speaking to a 911 operator regarding her father, who seems almost comatose and unresponsive. The operator asks, "Is he unconscious, bleeding, injured?" The girl answers no to each of the questions, but responds that her dad is depressed. It illustrates that depression—as well as anxiety—is a serious issue that can affect one's thoughts, feelings, behavior, and overall physical health. Awareness is increasing throughout our society as we find more and more that some people who seem perfectly healthy are troubled by these disorders.

Anxiety is a normal reaction to stress. It's normal to feel anxious or worried at times. Everyone does. In fact, a moderate amount of anxiety can be good. It helps you to respond appropriately to real danger, and it can help motivate you to excel at your activities.

Typically, anxiety goes away when the triggering event is over. However, anxiety is a problem when it becomes an excessive dread of everyday situations. People with anxiety disorder experience excessive fear and worry that are out of proportion to the situation.

Causes of Anxiety and Depression

There's no exact scientifically proven cause for depression or anxiety. The debate will probably rage forever as to the role of environmental factors versus genetics; the conditions likely result from a complex interaction of both.

Depression and anxiety often run in families, yet not everyone with a family history will develop them. Similarly, many people with no family history of these disorders can succumb to them. Experts believe that chemical imbalances in the brain's neurotransmitters are related to both anxiety and depression, but there is no agreement as to whether changes in neurotransmitters are a cause or result.

Some of the factors that contribute to a tendency to depression and anxiety include:

- Stress
- Heredity
- Alcohol and drug abuse. Although drugs are often cited as ways to ease depression and anxiety in the short term, many believe that these substances contribute to both depression and anxiety in the long term.

Regular exercise and taking time to relax are two of the healthiest activities you can do to help cope and sometimes control these experiences. There are many successful stories of Thai Yoga Massage helping people manage and even come out of anxiety and depression. This is mainly due to the deep spirit of metta, or loving-kindness touch, in the practice, but massage is only one part of a broader plan. Most important is to seek professional help when experiencing prolonged depression and anxiety.

THAI YOGA MASSAGE TREATMENT

ANXIETY AND DEPRESSION CASE STUDY

Recipient: Matt Shanle

Age: 31

Sex: Male

Height: 5'7"

Weight: 145 lbs.

Occupation: Lab technician

Presenting Issues: Anxiety, depression

History: Works mostly in isolation conducting experiments on rice cultures. Working conditions include poor fluorescent lighting. Has fought depression on and off for ten years. Recently also feels high anxiety and has begun making lists throughout the day, as he continually has a nagging feeling he has forgotten to handle things that need his attention.

Is a very light eater, mostly restaurant food and easy-to-prepare meals at home. Drinks alcohol regularly, in part to help numb his anxiety. Notices that it helps temporarily but comes back worse the next day.

Massage Approach
Posture Customization

- Full-body general massage with the intention to boost the spirit and raise the energy level.
- Lots of vigorous sweeping should accompany postures to help break up stagnation.

Sen Lines

- Kalathari, Ittha, Pingkhala, Sumana

Ayurveda

- Pitta build, vata imbalance (Anxiety points to the need for a vata-decreasing massage.)
- Pace: Moderate
- Pressure: Firm, but not too strong
- Postures: Balance of spinal twists, forward bends, backbends
- Vayus: Prana, Vyana
- Marma points: Amsa, Adhipati, Sthapani

Contraindication

With a vata imbalance and a partial goal to help boost the energy level, focus on Prana Vayu to bring more vitality into the body, Vyana to circulate energy, and sen lines and chopping to clear blockages. Postures can be firm but not too strong, so as not to aggravate vata.

Lifestyle Approach

Yoga Routine Recommendations

- Three Sun Salutations
- Standing twist, such as Triangle
- Mountain pose
- Five-minute relaxation

Food Recommendations

- Nurturing foods, home-cooked meals
- Reduce or eliminate alcohol
- Stews, soups, khichuri
- Whole-grain breads
- Some fish
- Organic foods when possible

Lifestyle Recommendations

- Keep good company with people who inspire you.
- Consider changing labs to one with more human interaction.
- Routine exercise practice: walking, yoga, swimming.
- Receive regular Thai Yoga Massage.

PUTTING IT ALL TOGETHER:
60-MINUTE THERAPEUTIC MASSAGE FOR ANXIETY AND DEPRESSION

Posture	Book*	Page #	Notes
Sitting Postures			
Namaskar	3	70	
Palming Shoulders	3	71	
Rolling Pin	1	61	
Lunar Stretch	2	91	
Shiva Twist	2	92	
Shakti Twist	2	93	
Row Boat	1	69	
Prayer Pose	1	70	Extended sweeping, chopping, Amsa marma, squeezing shoulders
Foot Postures			
Thumbing Sen on Sole	1	77	Sen Kalathari
Plantarflexion	1	74	
Dorsiflexion	1	75	
Toe Arc	2	106	
Foot and Ankle Rotation	1	78	
Foot Spinal Twist	1	79	
Thumbing Sen on Dorsal	1	80	Sen Kalathari, Ittha, Pingkhala, Sumana, Toe Cracking
Milk the Cow	1	82	Extended sweeping
Single Leg Postures			
Palming/Thumbing Sen	1	84	Sen Kalathari
Tree	1	88	
Nataraj	2	114	
Side Kick	1	91	
Single Leg Extension: palming	3	96	
Back Postures			
Back Massage	1	111	Work all sen lines and many variations that reduce thumb work to work out tension in head, neck, shoulders, and back
	2	127	
	3	120	
Pillow Cobra	1	114	Finish with extended sweeping and light chopping
Double Leg Postures			
Half Plough	1	118	
Yoga Mudra	1	122	
Thai Lute	2	137	Extended stretch and shaking the legs
Abdomen, Arm/Hand/Head Massage			
Abdomen 1 Massage	1	125	
Arm/Hand/Head Massage	1	130, 135	Sthapani, Adhipati marma
Sitting Posture			
Namaskar	3	70	

*Book 1 = *Thai Yoga Massage*, Book 2 = *Thai Yoga Therapy for Your Body Type*, Book 3 = *Advanced Thai Yoga Massage*

After Treatment

It is recommended to have regular Thai Yoga Massage treatments as often as once a week.

A Word of Caution

While this treatment may prove to be effective, it does not replace medical advice from a doctor.

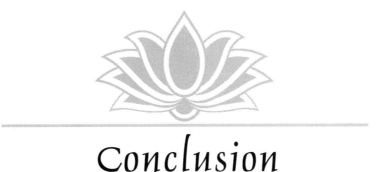

Conclusion

Massage is a traditional medical treatment in China, India, and Thailand. Many people who suffer from a wide range of common ailments will first go to a traditional massage healer who will help relieve their health issues. Over the past fifteen years I've seen how yoga has transformed the West, and this influence is ever-growing. It has changed the mindset of people for the better. I believe that in the near future we will see yoga, massage, Thai Yoga Massage, and many other alternative arts become a part of our mainstream medical system just like in China, India, and Thailand.

The power of human touch for healing has been far underrated in the West. Studies have shown that compassionate touch yields amazing, measurable results even in plants. A plant that is touched with love and respect and spoken to gently will thrive whereas one that is verbally mistreated and touched with negative energy will soon be in a pitiful state. Imagine how much healing we could achieve—of poor health and even conflicts—if we were all to touch each other with metta. Indeed, massage is the twenty-first century Buddha's medicine.

May you all have a good practice.

Classifying Muscle Trauma

Musculoskeletal problems come in many shapes and sizes. There are many possible ways of categorizing these problems. One way is to divide them into injuries and diseases. This distinction may be artificial because some diseases are a result of an injury, and vice versa.

Diseases of the muscles can include pervasive neuromuscular disorders, such as muscular dystrophy, dystonia, cerebral palsy, and multiple sclerosis; or autoimmune diseases, such as ankylosing spondilitis, rheumatoid arthritis, and other such diseases. While there is some clinical evidence about the benefit of Thai Yoga Massage in alleviating symptoms of these conditions, these diseases are extraordinarily complex and best tackled in conjunction with a trained physician.

Injuries of the muscles, tendons, skeleton, and articulations come in their own confusing variety of conditions, from meniscal tears to compound fractures, but for our purposes, it is probably best to divide them into two main categories: traumatic and chronic.

Traumatic injuries include breaks of the bone and trauma to the ligaments, tendons, muscles, bursa, cartilage, and other soft tissues of the body. Although we can work around a broken bone, this is not something we can treat in and of itself.

LIMITING THE INFLAMMATION RESPONSE IN MINOR TRAUMAS

The inflammation response is a normal part of healing that involves histamine release, vasodilatation, platelet action, leucocytes for cleaning, and collagen for scar tissue.

There is, however, an immediate stop valve for minor traumas. The body treats any injury as potentially life threatening, so you can speed up the healing process by limiting the inflammation response and adopting RICE.

Rest: Rest is important immediately after injury for two reasons. First, rest is vital to protect the injured muscle, tendon, ligament, or other tissue from further injury. Second, your body needs to rest so it has the energy it needs to heal itself most effectively.

Ice: Use anything icy to provide cold to the injured area. Cold can provide short-term pain relief. It also limits the inflammation response by reducing blood flow to the injured area. Keep in mind, though, that you should never leave ice on an injury for more than fifteen to twenty minutes at a time. Longer exposure can damage your skin. The best rule is to apply cold compresses for fifteen minutes, and then leave them off for at least twenty minutes.

Compression: Compression limits the inflammation response. Some people notice pain relief from compression as well.

Elevation: Elevating an injury reduces swelling. It is most effective when the injured area is raised above the level of the heart. For example, if you injure an ankle, try lying on your bed with your foot propped on one or two pillows.

SPRAINS

A sprain is an overstretch injury to a ligament. The cause of a sprain is a trauma-related sudden twist or wrench of the joint beyond its normal range of motion.

Acute Symptoms

Acute symptoms occur in immediate response to an injury and vary according to the severity of the sprain as follows:

Grade 1: Minor Stretch to the Ligament

- There is mild pain, local to the injury, at rest and during activity, stressing the ligament.
- Minimum local edema, heat, and bruising.
- The joint is stable.
- The client can continue activity.

Grade 2: Tearing of Some or Many Fibers of the Ligament

- There is a snapping noise and the joint gives way.
- The pain is moderate at rest and with activities that stress the ligament.
- Moderate local edema, heat, and bruising.
- Joint instability, if present, is slight.
- The client has difficulty continuing the activity due to pain.

Grade 3: Complete Rupture of the Ligament or a Fracture of the Ligament Attachment

- There is a snapping noise.
- The pain may be intense or mild at rest.
- Marked local edema, heat, and bruising are present.
- Hematoma may be present. Joint effusion may occur if the joint capsule is damaged. If blood goes into the joint space, a hemarthrosis occurs.
- Joint instability.
- The client cannot continue the activity.

In All Grades of Sprain

- The bruising is red, black, and blue.
- There is decreased range of motion local to the joint, as protective muscle spasm.
- Edema and pain limit movement.
- Depending on the severity, there is little, moderate, or severe loss of function of the affected joint. The joint may be taped, splinted, or otherwise supported. With a lower limb sprain, the client may use crutches. With a Grade 3 sprain, the ruptured ligament may be surgically repaired, then immobilized. Other structures compensate for this.
- A strain or contusion of the muscles crossing the joint, vascular damage, or nerve complications are possible with Grade 2 and 3 sprains.

Chronic Symptoms

Chronic symptoms persist over time and can be recognized by these signs:

- There is pain local to the ligament only if the ligament is stressed.
- The bruising is gone.
- Adhesions have matured around the injury.
- Hypertonicity and trigger points are present in muscles crossing the joint and in compensating structures.

- Full range of motion of the joint is restricted.
- A pocket of chronic edema may remain local to the ligament.
- The tissue may be cool due to ischemia.
- There is a loss of proprioception at the joint.
- The joint is unstable with a Grade 3 sprain unless it is surgically repaired. The joint may be immobilized for up to ten weeks after surgery.
- Muscle weakness or disuse atrophy may be present in muscles crossing the affected joint, particularly with immobilization.
- The client may need taping or elastic bandages for activities that stress the joint.

STRAINS

A strain is an overstretch injury to a musculotendinous unit. The causes of strain are a sudden overstretching of the muscle or an extreme contraction of the muscle against heavy resistance.

Acute Symptoms

Acute symptoms are in immediate response to a strain and vary in degree as follows:

Grade 1: Minor Stretch and Tear to the Musculotendinous Unit

- Local mild heat or edema. Bruising may not be present.
- Some tenderness at the lesion site.
- Minimal loss of strength.
- The client can continue the activity with mild discomfort.

Grade 2: Tearing of Some or Many Fibers of the Musculotendinous Unit

- Snapping noise or sensation at the time of injury.
- Moderate heat, edema, and bruising at the injury site.
- A gap may be felt in the tissue.
- Moderate tenderness.
- Moderate pain with activities contracting or stretching the affected unit.
- Moderate loss of strength and range of motion.
- Difficulty in continuing the activity due to pain. Some disability of the activity on the following day.

Grade 3: Complete Rupture of the Muscle or Fracture of the Tendinous Attachment

- Bruising: red, black, and blue.
- A hematoma is present at the injury site.
- A gap can be felt in the tissue, and the muscle may be bunched.
- Severe pain at the lesion site.
- Immediate loss of strength and range of motion (ROM).
- The client cannot continue the activity.

Chronic Symptoms

Chronic symptoms persist over time and can be recognized by:

- The bruising is gone.
- Hypertonicity and trigger points are present in the affected muscle and in any compensating structures.
- Adhesions have matured around the injury.
- The tissue may be cool due to ischemia.
- There is discomfort local to the lesion site only if the muscle is stretched.
- With Grade 2 and 3 strains, the full range of motion of the joint crossed by the affected muscle may be reduced.
- If the ruptured muscle was not surgically repaired, there is reduced strength, since only the synergists of the affected muscle can function.
- Repeated strains result from overuse, usually from workloads that are too stressful for the muscle. Chronic inflammation results from overuse or from continuing to work an injured muscle. With repeated strains, a pocket of chronic edema may remain local to the injury site.

There is reduced strength of the affected musculotendinous unit and possible disuse atrophy.

TENDINITIS

Tendinitis is inflammation of the tendon. Tendinitis results from microscopic tearing of the tendon due to overloading. Inflammation results.

Symptoms

- ◆ Grade 1: Pain only after the activity.
- ◆ Grade 2: Pain at the beginning of the activity, which disappears during and reappears after.
- ◆ Grade 3: Pain at the beginning, during, and after. Pain may restrict activity.
- ◆ Grade 4: Pain with activities of daily living. Pain gradually worsens.
- ◆ With all grades, there is a gradual onset of inflammation, heat, and swelling along the tendon or the tendon sheath and decreased range of motion for the affected muscle.

BURSITIS

Bursitis is inflammation of the bursa (fluid-filled sacs that reduce friction where bones meet other body parts). The cause of bursitis is overuse of structures around the bursa causing excessive friction. It is usually a secondary result of a condition such as tendinitis. Muscle imbalance, poor biomechanics, postural problems, and inflexibility are contributing factors.

Symptoms

- ◆ The bursa is compressed and irritated by surrounding structures.
- ◆ Inflammation, heat, and swelling are present.
- ◆ Pain is deep and burning, at rest and during activity. Pain may disturb sleep.
- ◆ Pain may refer to places distant from the injury.
- ◆ Restricted range of motion of the affected joint.

Resources

THAI YOGA MASSAGE TRAINING

The Lotus Palm School, founded by Kam Thye Chow, is one of the first Thai Yoga Massage schools in North America to have our certification program recognized for practice as a base modality by professional massage associations, including the National Certification Board for Therapeutic Massage and Bodywork (NCBTMB).

Our instructors teach courses worldwide. Please consult our website for the most up-to-date teaching schedule. If you are interested in hosting Lotus Palm for a workshop in your area, please be in touch. In addition, Lotus Palm is now offering a unique opportunity for students to learn directly from Kam Thye Chow through online courses.

Lotus Palm School of Thai Yoga Massage
5244 St. Urbain
Montreal, Quebec
Canada H2T 1S5
www.lotuspalm.com
info@lotuspalm.com
(514) 270-5713

PRACTICE AIDS

The Lotus Palm School offers a complete product line of Thai Yoga Massage items to support and inspire your practice.

Lotus Palm Mat Set

The Lotus Palm mat set consists of the main mat and two portable side mats, enabling the practitioner to expand the width of the mat and offering easy access to the removable mats from either side. These mats are suitable for Thai massage, shiatsu, Phoenix Rising yoga therapy, Breema, and all forms of floor work.

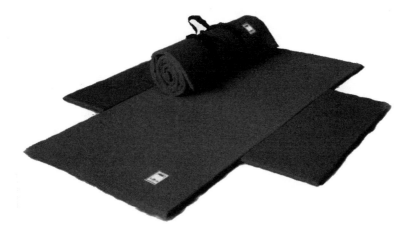

Other Products

Thai Yoga Massage book and DVD by Kam Thye Chow
Thai Yoga Therapy for Your Body Type by Kam Thye Chow and Emily Moody
Lotus Palm Music CD by Uwe Neumann
Handmade Thai pants specifically for bodywork
Sheets for the massage mat
Pillows for massage and prenatal Thai Massage
T-shirts
Meditation cushions

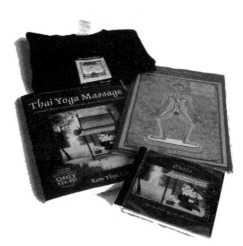

To order mats, books, DVDs, CDs, clothes, meditation cushions, and sheets:

info@lotuspalm.com

www.lotuspalm.com

(514) 270-5713

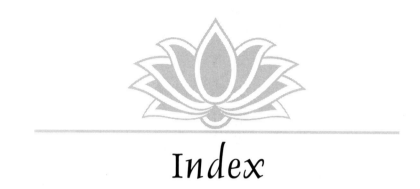

Index

Page numbers in *italics* refer to illustrations.